Humanity at the Heart of Practice

Humanity at the Heart of Practice:

A Study of Ethics for Health-Care Students and Practitioners

By

Beverly J. Whelton
and Jane Neuenschwander

Cambridge
Scholars
Publishing

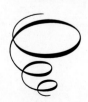

Humanity at the Heart of Practice:
A Study of Ethics for Health-Care Students and Practitioners

By Beverly J. Whelton and Jane Neuenschwander

This book first published 2019

Cambridge Scholars Publishing

Lady Stephenson Library, Newcastle upon Tyne, NE6 2PA, UK

British Library Cataloguing in Publication Data
A catalogue record for this book is available from the British Library

ISBN (10): 1-5275-3280-1
ISBN (13): 978-1-5275-3280-9

TABLE OF CONTENTS

Appendices

Introduction to the Text

Every semester, some students suffer the loss of a friend or family. This is a heartbreaking reality. Sometimes students will talk about their family's need to decide whether or not to take the friend or family member off life support. This is a complex decision. Questions include: Is there a designated health care agent and is there a written document of the person's wishes, often called a living will? Is there estranged family? Are there family members living far away? How long until they can arrive? What was the person's health prior to this event? What are the religious perspectives of the person and the family? In this difficult scenario, sometimes family members are confident and peaceful; sometimes they are anxious and irritable, but it is always a sad time. In the midst of this sorrow, life and death decisions must be made.

A Difficult Situation

An example of such a difficult situation was in the news in December 2013 following a California court decision to extend life support for Jahi McMath. The 13 year old girl hemorrhaged after tonsillectomy surgery and went into cardiac arrest. She was resuscitated and put on a ventilator for life support. Three days later she was assessed as brain dead; having no central nervous system function.[1] Thus far, no one has recovered from brain death, so in all fifty states brain dead is dead. The person can be legally taken off of life support and their donated organs transplanted. Jahi's family did not accept this assessment. It is quite natural for her family to think of her as still alive. They could see her chest rise and fall with mechanical ventilation. Cardiac rhythm has been restored so the body has warmth. But, there is no detectable brain activity.

Jahi's mother, Nailah Winkfeld, believed death occurred when the heart and lungs no longer functioned, and prior to 1968, this was the standard of death. There became a serious clash between medical and parental perspectives. Since Jahi had been declared dead and physicians do not treat the dead, she could no longer stay in the hospital. Her body was

---

[1] (December 30) http://www.bbc.co.uk/news/world-us-canada-25552818 (accessed January 1, 2014).

to be turned over to the coroner and a death certificate prepared. Ms. Winkfeld refused to allow the ventilator to be turned off. As a compromise, Jahi's mother was convinced to accept the issuance of a death certificate in order to have her daughter turned over to her care on a ventilator. Now, with a death certificate, no medical facility could admit the child for care.[2] With the help of financial donors, her mother transferred the girl on the ventilator in a private jet to New Jersey; the only state in the United States of America which allows a parent to overrule this diagnosis on religious grounds. For a long time Jahi's exact location was not disclosed. On June 22, 2018, four and a half years later, Jahi died from complications of another surgery.[3]

Humans are Concerned with Good and Evil

Humans are the only beings in the world who are concerned with what ought to be done. Humans perceive the impact of another human's action as good or evil, moral or immoral. Health care is humans caring for other vulnerable humans and ethics evaluates the way humans treat each other so it is natural that this book about ethical decision making in health care uses humanity as its organizing structure.

Perceptions of the situation and what ought to be done are closely tied to one's values. These assessments and accurate expressions of the situation require self-knowledge, knowledge of the circumstances, inner strength, courage, and wisdom. There are issues of informed consent, surrogate decision makers, and distinctions between killing and letting die. These and other related issues, like the meaning of life and death, will be discussed in this text. In the First Section, we begin with the consideration of values and good reasoning. Philosophy is concerned with what can be known through the power of human reason, so we need to consider what it is to know, to grasp concepts and to use good reasoning to make arguments. In Section Two we discuss what it is to be a being in the world, which means we look at nature and then human nature. Section Three

---

[2] http://blackdoctor.org/484482/family-of-jahi-mcmath-say-she-is-healthy-as-beautiful-as-ever/2/ and
http://www.nj.com/somerset/index.ssf/2016/01/family_of_brain_dead_girl_sue_to_change_death_cert.html
[3] http://www.latimes.com/local/lanow/la-me-ln-jahi-mcmath-dies-20180628-story.html and "Jahi McMath's mother says she has 'no regrets' for keeping daughter on ventilator for years" by Samuel Chamberlain | Fox News.
http://www.foxnews.com/us/2018/07/03/jahi-mcmaths-mother-says-has-no-regrets-for-keeping-daughter-on-ventilator-for-years.html

considers persons, the professional and the patient. That will conclude the foundational content. Section Four moves to making good ethical choices and theoretical rules proposed by some philosophers to evaluate what the good choice is. Section Five provides issues at the beginning and end of life and concerns related to health care as a business. Although we will see examples of ethical concerns throughout the text the last three chapters seek to make clear some of the most challenging decisions.

Through the work of this course you will be able to (1) make decisions in moral situations by the application of principles of philosophical ethics, (2) understand the foundations of the philosophical principles you find compatible with your personal informal moral development, and (3) resolve ethical dilemmas into their essential components using a provided framework to make clear the conflicting values, policies, or principles to move to a principle-based solution. In order to communicate with fellow students, faculty and clinicians, you need the vocabulary of ethical conversations. Within this text, important terms appear in bold and are provided in the glossary.

SECTION ONE:

VALUES AND PRACTICAL REASONING

CHAPTER 1

VALUES

Objectives

Upon completion of Chapter One, you will be able to:

1. Describe the role of values in personal and community life.
2. Describe the role of values in ethical decisions.
3. Identify your core values and the principles that follow from them.

Introduction

If you are an undergraduate health-care student or clinical practitioner this book was written for you. It does not assume that you have already studied philosophy but uses philosophy for insight and instruction in making decisions in difficult situations. Philosophical activities assist in the development of clear thinking and careful decision making. Careful decisions lend to peaceful living, although sometimes the best we can do is reduce the tensions we have to live with. Being human is practically synonymous with seeking to be happy. Philosophy is a discipline that seeks to find the way to human happiness through understanding the world, especially human life. To a great extent, happiness is being at peace with your decisions.

You may be thinking, "*I do not care about some universal ideal called human happiness or what ancient philosophers have said about being happy. I just want to make decisions that keep me out of trouble. In fact, I never even think about my decisions. I just follow what I am told to do. I presume it is legal or I would not have been asked to do it.*" This book is very much opposed to this position. As a clinical practitioner, you must question. You are responsible for what you do and for doing the proper action within your health-care situation. This means that you must pay attention to the particulars of the situation and know what the reasonably intelligent practitioner would do.

Ethical Decisions are Similar to Clinical Decisions

Some ethical situations are not as clear as the clinical circumstances calling for decisions. Ethical decisions are similar to clinical decisions, though, in that one must know circumstances and principles that guide actions and apply a decision-making strategy to determine the action to be done. Ethical situations contain clinical information, but the decision is whether or not a particular action is the right or good in these particular circumstances. In both clinical and ethical decisions, the conclusion is whether or not the situation is a case of a known principle. In both cases, there can be a difference of opinion as to what ought to be done, but especially in questions of ethics because of differing positions on what is good for humanity based on one's values.

Community Values

In July 2002, the people of Quecreek, Pennsylvania, and the United States as a whole, focused attention and hundreds of thousands of dollars to rescue nine miners trapped 200 feet underground.[4] And yet, if one miner had needed a liver transplant it would likely not have been covered by his health insurance. How does this make sense? We are, thus, led to a deeply philosophical question, "What is justice and how can we have a just society?"

The scientist paleontologist in Australia, Dr. Michael Archer dreamed of restoring the extinct Tasmanian Tiger from alcohol preserved DNA fragments harvested from a one-hundred-year old museum specimen.[5] Other scientists strive to clone extinct dinosaurs[6] or prepare a cell that will replicate the constructed DNA.[7] Whether or not these projects are reasonable scientifically is one question. Ethically, one has to ask if this is a reasonable use of human resources and if these kinds of scientific activities ought to be done. Is it the case that something ought to be done, just because it can be done? Are there moral limits to be placed on science as a kind of human endeavor? Is it right to try to use dinosaur DNA to

---

[4] http://old.post-gazette.com/localnews/20020730money0730p3.asp. (last accessed July 30, 2018).

[5] http://www.petermaas.nl/extinct/speciesinfo/tasmaniantiger.htm. (last accessed July 30, 2015).

[6] http://weeklyworldnews.com/headlines/27557/scientists-clone-dinosaur/ (last accessed July 30, 2018).

[7] http://www.nytimes.com/2012/06/03/magazine/craig-venters-bugs-might-save-the-world.html?pagewanted=all#4. (last accessed July 30, 2018).

make new life if the funds were available? Aren't we morally free to use our money the way we choose? Is there a moral obligation involved in how we use our money? Ought the money to be reserved for a clear human benefit? Would it make a difference if the creature brought back to life was human? To a great extent, these are questions of meaning and value. An individual's answer depends on what he or she values.

Personal Values

Knowing your values, ethical principles, and clear reasoning can be especially important when you are working in a situation containing moral or ethical tensions. These tensions can occur when there is an emotional pull between right and wrong, or between two goods that cannot both be acquired, or two evils or discomforts that cannot be avoided. Knowledge and insight also help your decision-making in situations of ethical tension and in the stress of living with difficult decisions.

Ethical Dilemmas

These are situations in which arguments can be posed for doing two different things. There may be a conflict of values, policies, or principles so that one must determine priorities among them. A person can only do one of the two possible actions and once you have acted you cannot go back and undo what was done.

The most important skill you will gain from studies in philosophical ethics is to make principle-based decisions in complex situations that challenge you to ask, "What is the good that ought to be done?" In order to do this, we will consider personal and community values, the meaning of human life, the human good, individual and corporate virtue, principles from codes of practice, a just society, and the processes of ethical-decision making. Complex situations often have values, codes, and principles in conflict. The hallmark of an ethical dilemma is that once an action is taken, you cannot go back and make another decision. Dilemmas are resolved by careful identification and discarding of irrelevant details, analysis and selection of relevant content, determination of priorities, and identification of relevant principles and policies that support moral decisions and actions. Sometimes, what seems to be an ethical dilemma is actually a lack of communication and information. Then, once those involved know the particulars of the situation and the options, the action to be taken becomes clear, and the dilemma dissolves.

Management Decisions

When managers set a course of action they usually also set a time to evaluate that course of action, which is quite different from an ethical dilemma where one cannot reverse the action taken. If leadership is not satisfied with outcomes, the manager's program can be reversed, or one can alter the course of action. This is not so with health-care dilemmas. Someone might have already died, or the information is now known and cannot again be hidden. Again, you cannot undo what has been done. For example, if you, as the respiratory therapist, remove a patient from the ventilator as a terminal weaning, and the patient dies, you cannot go back and say, "No, I will not participate in this process." You already did. On reflection, you may think about whether or not this is an activity in which you would participate in the future, but you cannot undo your involvement or the current situation. As a clinician in healthcare, you will come to recognize an ethical dilemma, as distinguished from management, communication, and social problems, to name a few.

Common Moral Decisions

Unlike ethical dilemmas, daily moral decisions require little thought. Prior development and training from childhood prepares us to match situations and principles of acting well. However, in the resolution of ethical dilemmas, you need awareness of your values and foundation principles. Knowing yourself allows you to preserve your conscience while not imposing your views on other persons. Thus, your work begins with discovering your own values and principles that operationalize these values.

Seeking the Principle-based Action

Ethical inquiry and the quest for principle-based action take us to the beginnings of recorded Western thought. In Athens, Greece some 2300 years ago, Plato documented the arguments of his mentor, Socrates, in the dialogue play, *The Euthyphro.*[8] Euthyphro planned to take his father to court because Euthyphro's servant died, bound in a ditch, for killing the father's slave in a drunken fight. Euthyphro argued that the Greek gods

---

[8] The *Euthyphro* and *Apology* are in *The Collected Dialogues of Plato,* E. Hamilton and H. Cairns, editors. Princeton University Press, 1961, tenth printing, 1980.

would expect him to try his father for murder even though it violated Greek social norms or values. Since Euthyphro acted as if he knew what the proper action was, Socrates challenged him to provide the principles of just or right action. Although it is asked as a question, Socrates implied right action is not right because the community or a god says it is right. There is something in the behavior itself that makes it the right thing to do in a particular situation. Socrates is saying there are principles that can be known and applied.

Equality is a Principle

An early indication of equality among humans is found in Euthyphro's speech justifying his action. He argues the status of the person killed and one's relationship to the person who killed does not matter. A human death is a human death. The only question was whether or not it was justified. This was counter intuitive for a culture that had slaves, indentured servants, and other people in prejudiced positions (8b-c).

In *The Apology,*[9] Socrates argues that one must be free to ask questions, and to be a faithful citizen, a person is to challenge and to think for oneself. He would say students must be allowed to question interventions and challenge procedures. People must reflect on what they are doing, and have done, to discern the good and proper human action. This is what it is to be human. All of this questioning begins with oneself. Socrates' famous maxim from the conclusion of his defense in *The Apology* is, "The unexamined life is not worth living." (38a)

This text will return to consider principles and discovering principle-based actions, however at this time; we need to consider values and their impact on one's moral perceptions and selection of what is important. As soon as one evaluates the outcome of a decision, one's values become apparent. One's values point to acceptable outcomes from interventions and what is seen as an ethical principle for use in decision making. While we are free to determine our actions and to ask for respect for our conscience positions in support of our views, we need to be careful about sitting in judgment of another person's values. Nevertheless, it is necessary to discern when values and personal decisions can lead to benefit or harm. It is easy to say decisions leading to harm are not ethical, and they do not promote the human good. Yet we value many

---

[9] The *Euthyphro* and *Apology* are in *The Collected Dialogues of Plato,* E. Hamilton and H. Cairns, editors. Princeton University Press, 1961, tenth printing, 1980.

interventions that lead to both healing and harm. One example is the cures possible with chemotherapy. An oncologist spoke to me after a lecture once, and he was quite concerned. He firmly asserted that there was nothing he did that did not cause harm, but he did not like the implications that he was unethical. His hope was that the good of a potential cure outweighed the harm.

While health-care professionals may have opportunities to help people in crisis clarify their values, the professionals are not the ones to determine what the other person ought to value; neither should they impose their values. The professionals will clarify and inform but respect the other person's decision. But, this does not mean professionals assist in behaviors against their conscience or allow actions they know are harmful to the patient and other persons.

Later in this text, we will look at the foundations of some principles in order to strengthen our understanding and decision-making capacities. When there are different principles supporting different answers in the same situation, it is helpful to understand the origins and meaning of the principles in order to make a careful decision by prioritizing relevant principles. Since there are differences in ethical principles and your principles are selected from your values, it is helpful to begin a study of ethics with an understanding of yourself.

These few short paragraphs have suggested that to be an ethical practitioner it is important to know yourself and know your patients. You need to know yourself to avoid imposing your values on others. You need to know the patients' values in order to represent their needs and advocate for them. Additionally, it is very important to be aware of the values within your place of employment so you properly represent your employer. You need to know what you value and the principles you hold dear, so you can choose to work in an environment where people value what you value or at least respect your values. You have a conscience that needs to be respected, but you have an obligation to choose work in an environment whose mission and goals are at peace with your conscience.

Finally, when you come to know your patients, you enter their world and are better able to understand the meaning of what they say. Respecting your patients does not require that you affirm their life choices, but you need to see each patient as a fellow person, with a right to his or her values and personal choices. To enter the world of another, one must be aware of cultural, social, and religious preferences and expectations. Respect for the individual requires that one act in culturally sensitive ways. This awareness allows your actions, treatment instructions, and health information to be relevant and, thus, more effective.

Conversation Starters:
1. Support your reasoning that we, as a community, should or should not fund speculative scientific projects.
2. Describe examples of projects you would want the community to fund. Provide support for your projects.
3. What evidence is there that humans share common capacities requiring common treatment of people throughout the world?

Reflection Submissions:
1. Can one's cultural heritage lead to immoral actions? Provide an example where culture provides positive guidance then provide an example of culture not leading positively. By what standard (standards) did you make this evaluation?
2. Write a reflection sharing your ideas and experiences of situations in which values made a difference. Explain why you say what you say about the situations. Share your understanding of the connections between values and actions.

Outline for Chapter 1: Values
A. Introduction
B. Ethical Decisions are Similar to Clinical Decisions
C. Community Values
D. Personal Values
    1. Ethical dilemmas
    2. Management decisions
    3. Common moral decisions
E. Seeking the Principle-based Action
    1. Equality is a principle

Terminology for Chapter 1
Moral or ethical tensions
Dilemmas

CHAPTER 2

PRACTICAL REASONING

Objectives

Upon completion of this chapter, you will be able to:

1. Distinguish between deductive and inductive reasoning; speculative and practical reasoning.
2. Apply the practical syllogism in resolving select ethical questions.
3. Use the normative ideals of Principlism: Nonmalfeasance, Beneficence, Autonomy and Justice as first premises in the practical syllogism.
4. Recognize the role in arguments of the principle of identity and the principle of non-contradiction.

Introduction to Arguments

While you can decide what ought to be done intuitively, based on how you feel, this is not as trustworthy as expressing reasons using language. Feelings are important indicators, but they are just indicators and not a solid base for decisions unless supported by reason. Developing sentences, expressing thoughts and feeling in words clarifies one's thinking. When you develop statements of values, beliefs, positions, principles and circumstances, you can form an **argument** that can then be thoughtfully evaluated for the support provided the conclusion. This support is by formal argument, which will be covered in Chapter Three. Assertions or affirmative sentences are **propositions.**[10] These propositions are claims that may be evaluated as true or false and offered as **premises** in support of another claim, the **conclusion** that an action ought to be done or not done.

Nuclear medicine students develop their skills through working with

---

[10] Watson, J.C. and Arp, R. Critical *Thinking: An Introduction to Reasoning Well*. New York: Continuum International Publishing Group, 2011, p. 34.

clinical preceptors in the hospital. It is my understanding that in some departments experienced practitioners give a slightly larger dose than in the protocol to increase absorption and decrease waiting time, so more patients can be processed in the allotted time. In this way, the department is on time and earns more money for the hospital. Some students experience ethical tension as they must decide if they ought to follow this practice and even if they ought to report this variance to a hospital administrator. It is a common practice but in violation of policy and may endanger the patient as it delivers a slightly higher dose of radiation.

An argument for compliance with this practice includes the propositions that it is common practice, experienced technicians do this, processing more patients makes the department look good and makes more money for the hospital. Each of these points is a propositions stated as a premise for the conclusion that the student ought to follow the same practice. This is an **inductive** argument. Each proposed reason provides more evidence that strengthens the case concluding to the behavior. On the other hand, the value of following policy and protecting patients from radiation argue **deductively** from general statements to the conclusion that the student ought not to give larger doses of radioactive dye.

Coming to Know Concepts

Before further considering principles and forming ethical propositions, it will be helpful to consider how we come to know our world on the conceptual or universal level. This involves ideas in our mind, and how these ideas (concepts) are related to what exists outside of the mind. From our experiences of the world, the intellect grasps similarities across items or settings. Through this capacity to grasp similarities and differences the intellect forms concepts. **Concepts** are general ideas. They cross time and place and are formed in the intellect as we experience individuals. When we think and talk and study we use concepts. They are also called **universals** because they leave aside the uniqueness of individuals to express what is common to the set of particular individuals that can be experienced. Concepts (universals) are expressed in words, that is, terms that can then be used to label other items of the same kind. On the simplest level, the sentences we speak use concepts expressed as nouns, adjectives, quantifiers, logical connections and so on. With the sentence, "The baby is hungry," the nouns 'baby' and 'hunger' are concepts formed in the intellect from experience of the world outside of the mind and labeled with the terms "baby" and "hunger." "The" is a quantifier indicating one, and "is" provides the logical connection. In this case "is" expresses the state of being or condition of the baby being hungry. The word "is" logically joins the subject and the predicate of the sentence. Logical concepts are drawn from the structure of the world but do not exist as items in the world as a baby does. One needs to be alert to the way words direct us to both concepts in thought and particulars in the world of experience outside the mind. The extra-mental reality of babies like, Betty and Joe, give rise to the concept that is then labeled with the term "baby." This labeled concept can then be used whenever such a being is experienced. This process allows us to know and to accurately speak about this world in which we live when the concept is accurately identified and labeled.

Mathematical Concepts in Measurement

When we measure blood pressure and other physical parameters these measurements are accurate within the capacity of our instruments and our ability to observe. Measurement is a way of increasing accuracy. The numerical properties can be separated from the physical. Blood pressures or blood sugars can be considered separate from the person with these readings. These measurements can then be compared to a chart of average readings and what they indicate, or they could be collected to graph this person's data as an indication of their bodily function. Errors can be reduced by repeated measurements and there is little debate about the meaning of the data.

Non-mathematical Concepts

With non-mathematical concepts, it is easy to misunderstand or misinterpret each other. Some ways we misunderstand are by faulty hearing, being distracted or by using the wrong word for a concept. We may also misunderstand another person when we think we already know what the other person means. Additionally, we interpret experiences differently because of our differing backgrounds but especially when anxiety or illness alters perception. With our tendencies to misinterpret, it is critical to confirm what the vulnerable person is meaning to communicate. As professional practitioners, we have an obligation to enter the patient's understanding, to ask and attend to their perception.

Concepts Build Arguments

The previous paragraphs have discussed the formation of concepts; mathematical and non-mathematical are drawn from the world of experience and imagination. Concepts can be formed into sentences having subject and predicate. The predicate is what is being asserted of the subject, it is thus making a claim that can be tested as true or false. These sentences asserted as propositional statements are the foundations of arguments. As provided above, an **argument** is a set of propositional claims, one claim is the **conclusion** being asserted, and the others are **premises** providing support for the conclusion. These propositional claims are the tools of communication useful in resolving ethical tensions and dilemmas. A syllogism is a set of three claims. The conclusion attributes the predicate content of the subject because of the relationships between terms within the two premises. A valid syllogistic argument follows the algebraic formula A=B; B=C; therefore A=C. B is called the middle term and connects A and C. The classic example is All men are mortal (capable of dying), Socrates is a man; therefore, Socrates is mortal. Being human is the common term that connects Socrates to mortality. If it is true that all humans are mortal (using more contemporary language) and if Socrates is a human and not your street name, then Socrates is Mortal.

Two Ancient Laws of Thought

There are two ancient principles in philosophy that impact reasoning and our work in ethics, the **principle of identity** and the **principle of non-contradiction**. According to Aristotle, the principle of identity says, "Whatever is is."[11] Expressed in this way the principle of identity is a **tautology,** that is, it cannot be false. It just is, but written this way, it tells us almost nothing. In another more important sense, the principle of identity is fulfilled when we accurately identify an object (or person) as the kind of being it is. The principle of non-contradiction says the same thing cannot both be and not be at the same time and in the same respect. Let's clarify these a bit further.

The Principle of Identity

There is an expression that says, "If it looks like a duck, walks like a duck and quacks like a duck, it is a duck."[12] This list of attributes, used to indicate the object in question, is helpful but insufficient. This is especially clear in today's world of technology. It is possible to have a mechanical

---

[11] Aristotle, *Metaphysics* IV, 4.
[12] *Cambridge Idioms Dictionary, 2nd ed.* Copyright © Cambridge University Press 2006.

duck which does each of these and yet is not the living being referred to with the term 'duck'. The principle of identity requires that the terms be used in a **univocal** way; the meaning is the same each time it is used.

The living duck and the mechanical duck share the term, duck, but the term has two different meanings. In this case the use of "duck" is **equivocal**. This change in meaning gives rise to the term **equivocation**. When the meaning of a term changes within an argument resulting in equivocation, there is no argument. The set of claims may be asserted as an argument, but the premises cannot support the conclusion.

Earlier it was said that the principle of identity cannot be false, it is just the assertion of what is, like the universal statement, "All trees are trees." Nevertheless, the grasp of a new concept is accurate or inaccurate; complete or incomplete, not true or false. This search for an organism is often the concern of scientists, like searching for the cause of AIDS or capillaries providing for circulation or shadows observed on the moon showing there are mountains on the moon. If one's grasp is complete, statements using the concept are more likely to be true. In addition to the discovery of new beings, there are times when it is essential to identify something as what it is. One example is when it is questioned if all beings with human DNA are human.

The Principle of Non-contradiction

The other ancient principle helpful in ethical argumentation is the principle of non-contradiction. "The same thing cannot both be and not be at the same time in the same respect."[13] Something either is or it is not. For example, you cannot be in class in West Virginia and on the beach in Florida. Either you are here or you are not here. Nevertheless, you could be in class physically and in Florida mentally. These are two different respects. Also, you could be in class today and in Florida over semester break. These are two different times. Our electronic devices allow us to be on different continents at the same time, but not in the same respect.

The useful meaning of the principle of non-contradiction is seen in an example from Chapter One where the DNA from the Tasmanian tiger can only be DNA from the Tasmanian tiger. It cannot also be canine DNA. It is either Tasmanian or it is not. It cannot be Tasmanian and canine, or Tasmanian and not Tasmanian. One has to question, though, if having the preserved inert materials of DNA are sufficient to say we have the DNA. The dynamic living force of life and function is missing. In Chapter Three,

---

[13] Aristotle, *Metaphysics* IV, 4.

we will look further at the matter/form unity of living beings. Keep in mind the question, "If having the material or the form of something means we have that item?"

Being Philosophical

Science is concerned with asserting hypotheses, testing, measurement, generalizations and supportable explanations. Caring for patients is an interpersonal process that can be deep and filled with meaning and feelings. Trying to understand patient care through research, based in measurement, seems incomplete and somehow shallow. Yet articles focused on description, opinion and ideas also seem insufficient. Contemporary research in health care uses both quantitative and qualitative methods determined by the question being asked.

From the time of Galileo to Isaac Newton, a hundred years later, there was a change in scientific inquiry away from verbal explanation and logical proofs to mathematical explanations and mathematical proofs. The history of science provides a time when questions were answered through understanding of concepts and argumentation. Interesting for our discussion, this tendency to question and the desire for answers is what it means to be **philosophical.** So, most of us are philosophical because we question. We all have a set of beliefs, a philosophy of life that guides the decisions we make. Philosophers openly ask what they believe and why they accept those beliefs or positions. They look for support for holding a certain position. What follows, in terms of behavior (actions done), if done thoughtfully is because one holds particular views.

In Chapter One, you were asked to consider what you hold as core values. When these values were united to the principles that follow from them you identified what could be your core beliefs. This is a good time for you to consider why certain values are important to you, and the actions you would take based on these beliefs.

Philosophers use experience, knowledge, careful thought, and the principles of reason (logic) to answer questions in a way similar to how contemporary scientists follow the logic of the scientific method, experiments, and mathematical analysis to answer research questions. In everyday life, we often ask questions about what something is, how it works, what we ought to do, how to get something done, or how to avoid being in trouble. Philosophers ask questions like, "What is it to be human? How ought humans to be treated? Are humans really free to choose their actions? If so, how do we know they are free? What evidence indicates we are free? What is the impact on personal and community living if we are free? Or, if we are not free, why do we feel like we are free?" Most of us consider these things a mystery, if we think about them at all. These questions are important because if we are to hold people accountable for their behavior, they must have been free to choose the action.

Metaphysic as a Division of Philosophy

Have you ever tried to figure out what is common to all that exists? The question itself tells us that existence is what is shared as common to all. This answer derived from the question may seem trivial. It is a tautology, but it is not trivial. There are reasons to consider the meaning of existence and the good of existence. The deepest thoughts are very simple, even profound. **Metaphysics** is the division of philosophy that searches into the origins and principles of existence. Some other questions that metaphysics considers include: (1) what can be known of existence within available evidence and human reason, (2) and what, if anything, can be known of highest being. This being is usually what is referred to when we say "God."

The Philosophy of Nature

The study of change or motion, common to all of nature, falls within the philosophy of nature. **Natural philosophy** is distinct from metaphysics in that it studies the changeable natural world, rather than all that exists or immaterial being. Specific sciences, like biology, chemistry and politics seek to understand their particular aspect of nature, be that the living cell, elements, or social structures. **Ethics,** as a natural discipline, is the study of the human person, as an individual acting within community. It is inquiry into how one ought to be treated and how one ought to act toward others.

Mathematics Used by Philosophers

Mathematics is reasoning with numbers and figures separate from material existent things. Since numbers and figures are abstracted from matter and idealized in the mind, results generated through purely mathematical operations are necessary and certain. In other words, the results are what they must be. For example, two plus two is four whether you abstracted the two from apples, cats, light years, or people. The formulae are persistent. Think of it! The Pythagorean Theorem is just as valid today as it was 2500 years ago.

Ethics is a Study of Proper Human Action

Metaphysics, natural philosophy, and mathematics are the three major divisions of philosophy, or knowledge. These were identified by Aristotle, the classical Greek philosopher and student of Plato. A significant impact follows from viewing ethics as a study of human action within the classical study of nature. This leads one to look within humanity itself for principles and causes of moral action [14](actions toward the human good). One impact of seeking principles within the nature of humans is found in the ways of nature. Nature acts for an end generally and for the most part. So, when principles are identified in nature, they are not absolutes like one might find in mathematics. Neither are they universally applicable as one might find with metaphysical principles of being, but they can still provide strong guidance within the complex circumstances of our lives in the world of change. These principles are stabilities that guide peaceful, happy living. Ethical principles are always applied within a context but not as arbitrary, blind rules. To say principles are used within a context does not mean that if a particular situation is an exception to the principle the principle is dissolved leaving us with no standards.

There is a need to know the principles and situations. One must carefully evaluate the fit between circumstances and principles. It does not damage the principle to make an exception, but it will probably make it more likely that we act contrary to that rule at a later time. In future chapters, we will consider principles, some of which are proposed as absolutes and some of which admit of exception. For our purposes, we need to be aware that ethics involves the careful identification, evaluation, and application of moral principles and rules of personal and professional conduct. All moral conduct is between persons within specific settings, that is, within a context. Principles can be proposed, examined, and discussed in an academic setting, but ethical (professional) and moral (personal) actions operationalize principles in particular, individual situations.

The Logic of Practical Reasoning

There is an identifiable pattern of reasoning that can be made explicit in the study of ethics. When known, it can be helpful in analyzing and

---

[14] It is not unusual to use ethical and moral interchangeably. Nonetheless, ethics most often refers to the study of moral behavior. Moral more often refers to personal codes, while ethical refers to professional standards and the actions of professionals.

responding to situations with ethical tensions. This is the logic of **practical reasoning**. A simple example is seen in the potential loss of a wallet belonging to the person walking in front of you. The wallet falls; you see the wallet and pick it up. Without hesitation, you tap the person on the shoulder and return his wallet. You may or may not have thought about keeping the wallet, but you did not keep it. We can infer that you saw keeping the wallet as a case of stealing because you could know whose property it was. As a child, you may have been taught that it is wrong to steal; stealing being defined as taking property with an identifiable owner and you are not that owner. The applicable principle or **moral maxim** is that, "One ought not to steal." The 'ought' is characteristic of a moral maxim. Practical reasoning inserts a moral principle within a situation requiring a decision of how one ought to act. The person seeking to do the right thing looks for a match between a known maxim and the circumstances with which he or she is being confronted.

Informally, practical reasoning depends on one's upbringing as the source of principles. When there is a maxim one learned in childhood, like do not steal, do not lie, etc., practical reasoning is simply a match, identification between the circumstances and the maxim. Keeping the wallet, in our example, would violate the known maxim or standard of behavior. Health-care practitioners add their disciplinary Code of Ethics and employment policies to their personal standards.

Study of Informal Logic

The discipline of Logic includes both this practical reasoning and more abstract forms of inductive and deductive reasoning. Logic is the tool of the intellect that prepares the mind for clear systematic thinking and for analyzing arguments. We now can state more formally from Watson and Arp, an **argument** is a set of statements or **claims**. One statement is the **conclusion**. The others are supporting content called **premises**. In uncomplicated situations of practical reasoning, the conclusion is that this is a case of a known maxim or principle. The maxim becomes the guide of what ought to be done. This reasoning is familiar within the clinical context as one's assessment concludes that the presenting situation is a case of a particular condition or diagnosis, which then prescribes the actions of the clinician. More complex situations require the development of arguments for what ought to be done. These arguments may be from principle to the situation in a **deductive** reasoning process or they may argue **inductively** from known cases. Grounded on prior principles from divine commands or philosophical analysis, deductive arguments assert "what ought to be done." Based on experience, inductive arguments are more probabilistic, resulting in what probably ought to be done, but allowing for unknown circumstances that could change the asserted conclusion.

An Example of Deductive Practical Reasoning

Given that nonporous materials block transmission of bacteria and viruses; it is required that all health care providers use gloves when in direct contact with patients (principle-premise). We are about to get patients out of bed for their walks (circumstances-premise), so we need to put on gloves (conclusion).

An Example of Inductive Practical Reasoning

The last five patients receiving IVP dye had adverse side effects. There is every reason to believe this person will also have a reaction to the dye. One is left to ask, "Do we have sufficient information to assert that the dye must not be used?" The answer is no, but we can say it probably ought not to be used or used with caution. To strengthen an inductive argument, you need additional information or appeal to principle. The first principle of action is, "Do no harm" (principle-premise). This situation could likely cause harm (circumstances-premise), so I will not use the dye (conclusion). Note both deductive portions of these arguments form practical syllogisms. A practical syllogism does not connect terms but principle and situation to conclude this is a case of the principle. From this one can conclude what ought to be done. The inductive argument above was strengthened by the addition of a deductive argument from principle.

Arguments Secure Decisions Not Actions

Academically, one might provide an ideal deductive argument with proper relationships between the concepts of the claims to make a **valid argument** and true premises that secure a **sound argument**. This is the very best support for the conclusion of what ought to be done, but sound arguments secure a decision; they do not secure human action. Humans are free to choose how they will act. Ethical principles are stated on a universal level but humans act within the world of particulars. Thus, we often do not grasp the application of the argument, or we may know what ought to be done but choose to do something else.

Even if one does argue effectively for what ought to be done, people are free to choose how they will act. There is a big gap between knowing what ought to be done and doing it. Aristotle argues that the actual choice is made at the moment of action and not in the decision of what ought to be done.[15] The knowledge of principles, circumstances, and a reasoned decision are required, but doing the good action also requires acting on the conclusion from reason about the issue or situation as opposed to acting on desire or fear. This ability to act on one's moral decision is the virtue of prudence or **practical wisdom**.

A Question of Justice as an Example of Ethical Reasoning

In another example of ethical reasoning, we could argue that justice is required and returning papers on time is a case of justice, so, returning papers on time is required as an application of justice. But, questions emerge in this more complex circumstance. What secures the premises as true? What makes us accept that justice is required or that returning papers on time is a case of justice? What is **justice**? What does it mean to say justice is required? Required for what? We could continue by asking what "on time" means. Are there exceptions and extenuating circumstances? To whom does the rule apply? In this way, we could argue about the premises and the application of the principle within a particular situation. Because moral reasoning generates questions, it may be difficult to secure a conclusion until all the questions are answered.

When confronted with a clear decision to act or not to act, to do either A or B, we use a **practical syllogism** as we did above with the wallet. To develop the circumstances of our more complex example, let's say a teacher has to decide whether to stay up late and grade papers, or return the papers late: late being after the two weeks, set by university policy. Because in our example returning papers on time is required to be just or fair to the students, this is a situation in which I need to stay up and complete grading the papers. On the other hand, 15 of the 25 papers still need to be graded and it takes 20 to 30 minutes a paper. Completing this project will take from 5 to 7 hours and it is already 7 pm. If this was your paper, would you want the teacher to rush just to complete the work and return the papers? No, it is also unjust not to give student work the attention it deserves. The students have worked hard preparing the papers. There is now a clash of two practical rules of justice; completing on time and giving the work proper attention. When taken apart and carefully

---

[15] Aristotle, *Nicomachean Ethics*, Book two. Translation and notes, M. Ostwald. Liberal Arts Press, 1962, 23rd printing, 1985.

analyzed, moral situations can be very complex. This clash of principles is a moral dilemma.

The format for moral reasoning in uncomplicated circumstances can be very practical. Given this situation and the principles accepted as truly binding on the teacher's action, one has to ask if this is a situation of a principle that ought to be followed. One may even reflect, given the particulars of the situation and the seemingly contradictory principles that are actively involved, which principle has priority? Conflicting principles lead to moral tension. Most moral errors happen when people do not see a principle (rule) as applying to them or when they do not see the situation as a case of the principle (rule).

As noted earlier, logic is the tool of all intellectual inquiry. It is intimately related to both the organization of concepts in the mind and language as the expression of those concepts and their relationships. Logic guides the discussion of our knowing the world and each other.

Two Levels of Logical Discussion

It is fairly easy to master the logic of good arguments, especially good practical reasoning. The difficulty is securing the truth of premises, or even accepting that the premises can be known. In moral reasoning, there are two levels of discussion. The first level accepts a principle as an assumption, an unsupported position that is obviously true from the meaning of the terms; sometimes this is called a first principle. From this first principle, one can work out what rules or practical moral maxims would follow. The second level of practical reason is the application of a principle or rule within specific circumstances and concluding that this particular circumstance is (or is not) a case of the rule that prescribes what ought to be done. The conclusion becomes that this situation is a case of the principle and I must act accordingly; or this situation is not a case of the principle and I am not required to act in the prescribed way. We recall that most practitioners have experienced this split between principles and actions before; we learn principles in the classroom and apply them in practice. In this way, practice is multifaceted. Clinicians require knowledge of principles and the ability to apply principles in situations. Academic testing of clinical questions and the learning of principles applicable to the discipline is the science of practice. Seeing the principles in clinical situations and adapting these principles for the needs of the specific patient is the art of practice.

Philosophical Answers and Normative Principles

The writings of philosophers have much to contribute to living a rewarding, healthy and robust life. As an example of the relevance of philosophy, consider the following ethical teaching of Aristotle who lived and wrote some 2300 years ago, as noted earlier. In our world of instant messaging, disposable goods, and microwave dinners, it is hard to imagine finding value in anything written so long ago. If you have ever given or taken a prescription you know the "five rights" of medication administration. Every health-care professional who administers medication has learned them. You may remember them as the (1) right medication to the (2) right person at the (3) right time in the (4) right amount in the (5) right way or mode of administration. Within Aristotle's ethical writings, *Nicomachean Ethics,* this ancient philosopher teaches that we are virtuous, acting with excellence, when we experience pleasure and pain "at the right time, toward the right objects, toward the right people, for the right reason, and in the right manner (1106b20-22)."[16] This is not bad advice either for taking one's medication or for peaceful living.

As a clinical practitioner, one is taught to act guided by principles and to make choices based on principles learned, and not just feelings or intuitions of what is needed in the situation. These feelings are important and tell us things that sometimes cannot be put into words but for the most part we are to (1) know what we are doing, and to (2) choose to act for the benefit of those served to move them toward the good end of health or a peaceful death, and we must (3) act consistently for the benefit of the patient and/or their family. These are also Aristotle's characteristics of a virtuous act (*Nicomachean Ethics* 1105a30-33). These readings suggest that clinical practice is an ethical practice. Health care professionals in all of the disciplines need to know discipline specific knowledge and skills, and to know about communications, organization, and building relationships, but they also need to be able to make decisions, and act for the good of others.

Normative Principles

Where do health care professionals find ethical principles to enlighten their thinking about ethical dilemmas? This focus on principles understands ethics to be **normative.** The position that each situation is open to its own interpretation and there are no common principles is called

---

[16] Aristotle, *NE*, Book Six.

relativism. Nonetheless, to assert that "each situation is open to its own interpretation" or that "there are no principles" asserts two principles contradicting the original statement. To assert there are no principles is to assert a principle. In many cases the promoter of relativism is not saying there are no principles but that not enough attention is given to individuals and their circumstances.

Nonetheless, this text seeks normative principles to assist with practical reasoning within moral situations. As was said **practical reason** sees circumstances and recalls a principle or maxim from earlier training. The conclusion drawn from practical reasoning is that this is a situation of the principle, or it is not an occasion of the principle. To add to the examples given we can consider our own studies. Offered the opportunity to view a copy of the exam a virtuous student will say "no" because it is a case of cheating. He or she was taught not to cheat because it is stealing. As stated earlier the maxims learned in youth resolve most moral situations. Within professional ethics there are some principles that have become moral ideals and are valued in themselves. They are as follows: (1) **Nonmaleficence,** or doing no harm, (2) **Justice** in distribution of goods and services, (3) **Autonomy**, which is a respect for person's self-determination, and (4) **Beneficence,** or doing the long-term good for the patient and community. Doing no harm is the minimum moral standard and is often captured as acting within the law. To be a member of the community, one can at least obey the law. Doing the good is a much higher standard calling for a different outlook. We cannot force others to do the good, but as professionals this is expected of us. Justice and autonomy can be seen as ways of achieving this good (A position developed and promoted by T.L. Beachamp and J. F. Childress).[17] These facets of an ethic called **Principlism** seem to stand alone. They are ideals to be preserved reminiscent of Platonic Ideals. In fact, in the writings of Plato, Justice is the primary ideal of human action leading to a harmony of the soul that is a happy, peaceful inner life.

Principles within Humanity

Practical normative principles may also be found from within what it is to be human, where principles like the ideal of Beneficence could be said to emerge prior to humanity. Principles from within humanity would consider what it is to be human. What are the unique human capacities?

---

[17] Beauchamp, T.L. and J. F. Childress, *Principles of Biomedical Ethics,* 6th Edition. Oxford University Press. 2008.

Philosophers down through the ages have asserted with some variation, that humans are unique in our capacity to know and to choose. To know is to have the truth. If you do not have a grasp that corresponds to what is actually the case, you do not know, you are in error. When we choose among options, we select what is perceived to be good. It may only appear to be good and not actually be so, but it was chosen as good (even if this was to steal or kill). In this way, one can say decisions that preserve truth and goodness are from within the meaning of human life. This reasoning provides what Thomas Aquinas calls the First Principle of Practical Reason: do good and avoid evil.[18]

Human Dignity

Dignity is a principle from within humanity but also from within one's community. My old, dusty, stained Funk & Wagnall's Dictionary tells me that to have **dignity** is to be stately, noble, worthy, excellent. I can see these attributes in the redwood, in the giraffe, and even in the monarch butterfly, but one has to ask, can these attributes really be found in humans so capable of crime and destruction? And yet, it is the value and dignity of each human life that leads hundreds, even thousands of individuals, to protest at abortion clinics and to march on Washington, D.C. each January. The unborn child may be severely disabled and require millions of community dollars to support their lives, and yet these protesters rejoice if one child is saved. The child could become a murderer or a great scientist, it is unknown, and yet they rejoice. How can this be? What is it that these protesters see? Many equally intelligent people would say that sacrificing the unborn is preserving the dignity and autonomy of the pregnant woman. And yet many of these women suffer such pain, remorse, and loss of their self-respect after an abortion. Is self-respect dignity?

Inherent Human Dignity

What is human dignity? Can it be given or destroyed? Although, individual humans can be valued or destroyed can the dignity of the individual be taken by another? Can we act in ways that destroy our own dignity? Some would say the sexually promiscuous and the prostitute do. And yet, the day laborer does not destroy his or her dignity. Their use of their bodies to care for themselves and their family are appreciated. What is the difference?

---

[18] Aquinas, *Treatise on Law. Summa Theologicae, Question 90-97.*

The Eighteenth-Century philosopher, Immanuel Kant, wrote that everything has either a dignity or a price.[19] There does seem to be something different in our relationship to a forest if we clear the underbrush to prevent a massive fire or if we clear the land in a business venture to sell the timber. We talk about live human organ donation as a very great gift, enhancing regard for the donor and preserving the life of the recipient. Currently, in America, the selling of organs is forbidden. Why? Some people need the money more than their kidney, which seems extra since we have two. The seller gets the necessary money that provides for their livelihood or a child's medical care and the recipient has another opportunity to live. Seems like good business, but, does this selling of body parts distort human dignity and the meaning of being human? One might say an individual is so much more than body parts that it is impossible to impact their inherent worth in this way. Others hold that any buying and selling of humans reduces them to a commodity. They even invoke visions of slavery. Is human dignity our inherent worth? Inherent means the value existing from within. Can we receive it and give it away? Can we really lose it?

Socially Attributed Dignity

Do all humans have the same value? If value is contribution, it seems not. The physician contributes more than the coffee vender, but is the physician as an individual human of greater value? And, even if this were the case, isn't their individual dignity equal? The Declaration of Independence holds we are created equal. Is this referring to our dignity? So many unanswered questions and yet, it seems we can manifest the dignity of our lives through living with nobility and excellence. There is an important difference between inherent dignity and socially attributed dignity. Inherent dignity is ours from the kind of being we are, capable of reason, freedom, and choice. Socially attributed dignity is our worth based on what we do, how we see ourselves and how we are seen by others. This is the dignity that is gained and lost. The murderer forfeits socially attributed dignity, not inherent human dignity, even though what was done was inhumane.

---

[19] I. Kant, *Grounding for the Metaphysics of Morals.* Translated by J.W. Ellington. Indianapolis: Hackett Publishing Company, 1981.

Conclusion

This chapter has introduced arguments, inductive, deductive and practical. We explored coming to know concepts because concepts form the subject and predicates of propositions. Awareness of concept formation impacts our thinking whether or not we can know the world as it is. Concepts are also called universals because they leave aside the uniqueness of individuals to express what is common to the set of particular individuals that can be experienced. Concepts are expressed in words that are terms that can then be used to label other items of the same kind. Measurement increases accuracy of data experienced and can lead to greater understanding.

Additional understanding of knowledge and language formation is found in the Principle of Identity and the Principle of Non-contradiction. Understanding of our world also requires the scientific method and philosophical reasoning. Divisions of Philosophy were articulated by the ancient classic philosopher Aristotle, Metaphysics (questions of immaterial being), Mathematics (abstracted from material being and now immaterial), and Philosophy of Nature (matter in motion). In this scheme, Ethics is the study of humans acting within community. That is, how humans ought to be treated and how they ought to act. Ethical principles are applied within a context but not as arbitrary blind rules.

There is an identifiable pattern of ethical reasoning called practical reasoning. The first premise is a guiding principle of what one ought to do, the description of a situation, and a conclusion, whether or not this principle is applicable in the current situation. The discipline of Logic includes this practical syllogism, and rules of inductive reasoning and deductive reasoning. Practical reasoning parallels clinical reasoning with identification of diagnosis and actions that follow on the diagnosis.

Even if one does argue effectively for what ought to be done people are free to choose how they will act. Acting on what one knows ought to be done is the virtue of prudence (practical wisdom). When principles clash, each advising a different action, one has a moral dilemma. Practice is multifaceted. Clinicians require knowledge of principles and the ability to apply principles in situations. Academic testing of clinical questions and the learning of principles applicable to the discipline is the science of practice. Seeing the principles in clinical situations and adapting these principles for the needs of the specific patient is the art of practice.

This text seeks normative principles to assist with practical reasoning. In addition to common moral maxims like, do not steal, professional ethics uses principles that have become moral ideals and are valued in themselves. They are as follows: (1) Nonmaleficence, or doing no harm, (2) Justice in distribution of goods and services, (3) Autonomy, which is a respect for person's self-determination, and (4) Beneficence, or doing the long-term good for the patient and community. Principles may also be found from what it is to be human with the capacities for knowledge and choice. Aquinas identifies the First Principle of Practical Reason as do good and avoid evil.[8] Dignity is a principle from within humanity but also from within one's community. Dignity divides into a person's inherent dignity as human and their attributed dignity as a member of the community.

Conversation Starters:
1. How does one learn what another person values? List some values which make a difference in how people are treated?
2. Share, with a classmate, a situation that you experienced or heard about where patients and practitioners had contrasting values. How did you (or they) work with their differences?
3. Use examples and arguments to support or refute the position that respecting human dignity is the normative principle for how we ought to treat people? You will need to begin by providing what you think "respecting human dignity" means.

Reflection Submissions:
1. Write a practical syllogism to resolve a situation of moral tension. Do this as if you were the one who needed to act.
2. Find an ethical dilemma in the news. Identify premises and conclusions used by the author to construct his position. Would this argument convince you to accept the author's position? Why/Why not?
3. Explain the following distinctions: (a) clearing land to prevent fire or clearing land to build a new theater, (b) donating an organ or selling it. In what way(s) does asking these questions vilify business?
4. Considering the above situation of the nuclear medicine student, if this were you, would you provide the extra radioactive medium? Would you report the situation, and if so, to whom would you say something? Explain your answers and use an argument to support each answer.

Classroom Activity in Argumentation:
1. With another student, develop a compelling (strong) inductive argument and a sound (valid arrangement and true premises) deductive argument for or against one of your favorite discussion topics. Examples of such topics include: freedom of speech, gun control, use of controlled substances (alcohol under age 21 or cigarettes under age 15), etc.
2. Join with another set of students and share arguments developed for #1 in this section. Look for where the premises could be improved. Notice that the focus is not on resolving the debate, but rather evaluating the arguments. Rewrite arguments to be as strong or sound as possible. That is to say, so the content of the premises is true and the relationships between the premises and conclusions are clear. If the arguments already seem strong or sound develop a rationale to support that position.

Outline for Chapter 2: Practical Reasoning
A. Introduction to Arguments
B. Coming to Know Concepts
    1. Mathematical concepts
    2. Non-mathematical concepts
    3. Concepts build arguments
C. Two Ancient Laws of Thought
    1. The principle of identity
    2. The principle of non-contradiction
D. Being Philosophical
    1. Metaphysic as a division of philosophy
    2. The philosophy of nature
    3. Mathematics used by philosophers
    4. Ethics is a study of proper human action
    5. The logic of practical reasoning
E. Study of Informal Logic
    1. An example of deductive practical reasoning
    2. An example of inductive practical reasoning
    3. Arguments secure decisions not actions
    4. A question of justice as an example of ethical reasoning
    5. Two levels of logical discussion
F. Philosophical Answers and Normative Principles
    1. Normative principles
    2. Principles within humanity
    3. Human dignity
    4. Inherent human dignity
    5. Socially attributed dignity
G. Conclusion

Terminology for Chapter 2
Argument
Propositions
Premises
Conclusion
Inductive argument
Deductive argument
Concepts
Universals
Conclusion
Premises
Tautology

Univocal
Equivocal
Equivocation
Philosophical
Metaphysics
Natural philosophy
Ethics
Practical reasoning
Moral maxim
Claims
Inductive
Deductive
Valid argument
Sound argument
Practical wisdom
Practical syllogism
Normative
Relativism
Nonmaleficence
Justice
Autonomy
Beneficence
Principlism
Dignity
Inherent dignity
Attributed dignity

SECTION TWO:

PHILOSOPHICAL PERSPECTIVES OF NATURE AND HUMAN NATURE

This section provides content for understanding why moral conduct is an issue in our lives. It answers big questions like: Can humans have truth of our world? What is it to make decisions and act in ways that express our humanity versus capacities we share with animals? This section develops human nature as the foundation for ethical practice as opposed to popular opinion and culture. It describes humans as individuals and as individuals in community. The next section, Section Three, considers humans as professionals and as patients.

CHAPTER 3

FOUNDATIONS OF KNOWING NATURE AND HUMAN NATURE

Objectives

After studying this chapter, you will be able to:

1. Distinguish between natural beings and artifacts of human life.
2. Describe the matter/form unity of natural beings, including humans.
3. Distinguish between natural and artificial interventions in healthcare.
4. Recognize valid and invalid formal argument forms.
5. Describe the relationship between the form as concepts in the mind and the form in items outside the mind that allows us to know the world.

Philosophy of Nature

Seeking a Stable Source of Moral Guidance

Some ask why one would study the Philosophy of Nature in a text about proper human action. The short and obvious answer is that many people do not believe it is possible to have knowledge of what it means to be human, and this book proposes to provide principles of behavior grounded in knowledge of human nature. If we cannot use experience and reason to know our world, our quest for natural principles of human action is futile. This does not deny either the complexity of life or the difficulty of coming to knowledge as opposed to belief. Neither does it reject the importance of socially constructed positions. The majority view is very important, especially in consideration of community resources. Sometimes the contemporary popular view would be considered wise from a philosophical understanding of human life, but sometimes popular opinion clashes with wisdom grounded in knowledge of being human. Can I be so bold as to say, a decision grounded in a philosophical understanding of human life is more secure than one which is popular because popular opinion and culture vary widely. This presumes we are able to make distinctions between being popular and being right. We are left with the questions, "What is right? What is good?"

Other Sources of Moral Guidance

Religious views provide guidance for many people, but requiring religious foundations for an action to be moral is unsupportable because we find there are people of good will everywhere who are without religious foundations, who have rejected these foundations, or even have rejected the existence of a designer and creator of the universe. Yet, these "non-believers" can act with moral goodness that promotes the human good. Thus, we argue that moral principles required for practical moral reasoning are accessible to the reasonably intelligent person. Nevertheless, we will agree with the classic Greek philosopher, Aristotle that students of ethics need to have moral training as a child in order to recognize moral principles and to have the virtue (wisdom and courage) to act on decisions from principle. He thought ethical actions begin with the actions we do as children under the guidance of our parents.[20] Even though family may be defined more broadly today as parental figures or role models, the necessity to train children remains. Recall parents giving the child a quarter to put in the offering plate or the Salvation Army bucket at Christmas or the requirement that the child share his or her toys. This is early training in the virtue of generosity.

Moving to the Knowledge of Human Nature

It is being argued that knowledge of what it is to be human can thus, provide principles that explain and at some point, prescribe the best or proper human actions to achieve the human good. This knowledge of humanity is universal and abstract. This is not knowing a particular individual or what they will do. Awareness of human freedom of choice is part of what is known and distinctive of humanity not just of individuals.

. If this coming to knowledge of nature is not possible, we would still know how to treat each other from cultural norms, the law, professional

---

[20] Aristotle, *Nicomachean Ethics.* Translated with and Introduction and Notes by Martin Ostwald. Indianapolis: Bobbs-Merrill Educational Publishing, 1962, Twenty-third Printing, 1985. Book 1, Ch. 3. pp. 5-6.

and religious standards. Nonetheless, considered as a global community, all of these vary. If we could come to knowledge of ethical norms from our knowledge of being human, we would have a more secure standard by which we could evaluate other proposed more variable standards.

Forms of Logical Reasoning

Given your values development and upbringing in virtue, it is possible to increase your moral sensitivity and acquire principles that can be applied in contemporary clinical settings within the practical syllogism. You may not have thought of yourself as having a moral upbringing. Nonetheless, if you did not, you would not have the patience, perseverance, courage, and wisdom (virtues) required to pursue your education.

Valid Logical Forms of Reasoning

At this point we need some Formal Logic[21] to develop critical thinking and show reasoning that supports one can know the natural world and following on that, what it is to be human. With the hypothetical statement "if…then," the "if" portion is called the **antecedent (p)** and the "then" portion, the **consequent (q)**.

Modus Ponens

What follows is a sequence of valid logical reasoning using the above hypothetical form of **Modus Ponens** [if p, then q: and p, therefore q]:

1. If humans are able to grasp stable generalizable content of items experienced in the world (p), then humans are capable of knowing the world (q): [if p, then q]
2. And, it is shown that humans can grasp stable generalizable content from items experienced in the world (p), therefore humans are capable of knowing the world (q). [and p, therefore (or so) q]

Extending the argument to the next sequence:

3. If humans can know the world (the above consequent (q) becomes

---

[21] Watson, J.C. and Arp, R. Critical *Thinking: An Introduction to Reasoning Well.* New York: Continuum International Publishing Group, 2011, p. 157.

the antecedent (p), then they can know what it is to be human (the new consequent).

4. And, humans can know the world, so they can know what it is to be human.

Using the valid deductive argument form, Modus Ponens, we have shown that it is possible to know what it is to be human. In a valid formal argument, if the premises are true, the conclusion must also be true.

Modus Tollens

The prominent philosopher of science, Karl Popper,[22] did not accept that knowledge advances through experience and inductive verification of theories, which he called conjectures. He argued that we cannot sufficiently verify our ideas because our observations are always within a particular world view. Nonetheless, we can falsify them. It only takes one contradiction to falsify the statement that "all p are q" or "all students are hard-working." The value of falsification in advancing knowledge led to the use of null hypotheses in social science research. A null hypothesis says there will be no significant difference between two variables in an asserted statement, hypothesis. Two important aspects of a null hypothesis follow: (1) "The null hypothesis (H_0) is a hypothesis which the researcher tries to disprove, reject or nullify." (2) "The 'null' often refers to the common view of something, while the alternative hypothesis is what the researcher really thinks is the cause of a phenomenon."[23] Consider that your graduate research is to prove the positive effect of an intervention on pain. You would assert that your intervention makes no statistically significant difference. Data collected may show that it is not true that there was no significant difference. By way of rejecting the null hypothesis, the research has shown your intervention was effective.

This reasoning process uses the other valid formal argument form of **Modus Tollens** [if p, then q: and not q, therefore not p].

1. If intervention p is not effective against pain (p), then there will be no significant difference between groups with and groups without intervention p (q): [If p, then q]

---

[22] Karl Popper, *Conjectures and Refutations*: The Growth of Scientific Knowledge. London, Routledge, 1963. A very helpful discussion of Popper and his work can be found at https://plato.stanford.edu/entries/popper/

[23] https://explorable.com/null-hypothesis

2. And, there was significant difference between groups with and groups without intervention p (not q), therefore intervention p was effective (not p). [and not q, therefore not p]

The negation of negative p and negative q is a positive result, rejection of the null hypothesis and acceptance of the researcher's desired result, showing their intervention was effective.

Invalid Logical Forms of Reasoning

Invalid argument forms are called **fallacies.** They look like secure arguments following the valid formal arguments, Modus Ponens and Modus Tollens, but are not. The argument might still be compelling when several premises, from different aspects converge or when similar results from multiple studies are added together, but they lead to probable results. They do not secure the conclusion.

The Fallacy of Denying the Antecedent

Often confused with Modus Ponens, the fallacy of denying the antecedent follows: If it is raining (p), then you will take your umbrella (q), it is not raining (not p), so you will not take your umbrella (not q). [If p, then q: and not p, so not q] The problem is it may rain later, so you will take your umbrella now.

The Fallacy of Affirming the Consequent

Often confused with Modus Tollens, the fallacy of affirming the consequent follows: If it is raining (p), then you will take your umbrella (q), you did take your umbrella (q), so it must be raining. [If p, then q: and q, therefore p] The problem is you may have taken the umbrella for a later time, and it is not now raining. It is awareness of this fallacy that leads most scientists to say they do not come to knowledge, just probability with their research. Consider the following: If the AIDS syndrome is caused by a virus, then infected serum after flowing through a micropore filter will still cause the AIDS syndrome. Serum after processing through a micropore filter still causes AIDS, so the AIDS syndrome must be caused by a virus (the fallacy). Actually, the researcher would say, it is possibly caused by a virus. After a great deal of testing, the scientists will say, it is probably caused by a virus. After they become convinced that if, and only if (**iff**), a virus has caused the syndrome would they get the results they have, scientists will claim the causal relationship.

The purpose in our consideration of these valid and invalid argument forms is to highlight that one can properly reason to principles of human practice. You gain insight into these principles when you combine your experience of what it is to be human, your philosophical inquiry into human nature, and careful reasoning. Many of us grew up with a given perspective on many ethical issues. The perspective was right because we were told it was. Now, you are being asked to decide for yourself, based on the nature of the action and its impact on the good of human life.

Knowledge of Nature

Nature as the World

Looking out the window, we see the flowers, grass, trees, maybe even fields and mountains or the beach. These are nature in the larger sense of the world around us. We may think we control our environment but then winds blow, the earth shakes or the water rises; we are called to remember that we are only a part of nature. In addition to nature as this world outside of the window or in the park, each person or thing has a **nature** that makes it be what it is. According to Aristotle, "Nature is a source or cause of being moved and of being at rest in that to which it belongs primarily, in virtue of itself and not in virtue of some concomitant [accompanying] attribute."[24]

Nature as an Internal Principle

We can contrast this sense of nature as an inner principle of development with the artificial or human-made. Natural things have their principle of change within them. Artifacts have undergone change from outside of themselves. They have been acted upon. The wooden desk can deteriorate because it is made of oak. It does not fall apart as desk, but as wood. Desks do not have internal principles of change, but when living the wood did have an internal principle of growth. The wood of the desk lacks this living principle and so the wood decays.

In this understanding,[25] nature is intimately indwelling and not something added to or associated with a thing, but what it is. This includes the living and the nonliving, the organic and the inorganic. One's nature gives rise to existence, growth and development, as well as one's

---

[24] 192b21-23 Translated by R. P. Hardie and R. K. Gaye, *Physica* in *The Basic Works of Aristotle,* Richard McKeon, editor. New York: Random House, 1941
[25] William A. Wallace, *The Modeling of Nature: Philosophy of Science and Philosophy of Nature in Synthesis.* Washington, D.C.: The Catholic University of America Press, 1996. p.158. Wallace was my major professor for my dissertation. I owe to him my understanding of the processes of nature and of knowledge. It would not be possible to reference sufficiently.

characteristic activities and properties. Using the concept of nature in this way comes from classical thinking, like the work of Aristotle and his medieval commentators. Existential and contemporary philosophers challenge this notion of stable natures or kinds of things. In fact, with all of the natural change we experience it does seem contradictory to say something remains the same. But there is stability in nature: the stability of the kind of being undergoing change.

Nature is the inner force which brings a thing to completion, and decline and decay are when it has reached the limit of size or existence. The elephant grows to a huge size compared to the ground hog, and lives much longer. These natural limits are within the animals and are set by the kind of animal they are. Nature generates these changes from within as when the sapling grows into a tree or the calf matures into a cow. Although the artist collaborates with nature, as when Michelangelo studied the marble before sculpting to ensure that it 'contained' the statue of David, the **artifact** has principles of change imposed on it. We generally think of artifacts as being made by humans. Even though the dam is an artifact of beavers and the nest of birds, philosophers reserve the term **artificial** for things made by humans. The principles of making a dam or nest were placed by nature within the beaver and bird; therefore, the dam and nest are **natural**. In contrast to humans, the animal is not choosing the shelter to build. It is written into the genetics of the species.

Natural and Artificial

The distinction between natural and artificial assumes new importance in the discussion of health-care interventions. Early practitioners like Florence Nightingale taught that the role of the nurse was to remove impediments so that nature could heal.[26] At the origins of formalized health care there were primarily physicians who focused on cures and nurses who focused on careful watchfulness, caring and hygienic practices. Today there are a great variety of health-care activities and disciplines. Even so, health care is care provided to humans by humans. For this reason, this text holds that humanity is the unity at the heart of health care.

Issues surrounding care for those in **Persistent Vegetative State (PVS),** require that one clarify their position on the artificial provision of food and fluid. It seems everyone must receive food and fluids from

---

[26] Florence Nightingale, *Notes on Nursing: What it is and what it is not.* New York: Dover Publications, 1969.

sources outside of themselves. What makes nutrition natural or artificial? What makes the provision of fluids natural or artificial? When the name changed from feeding to medical nutrition and medical hydration, did this change in name change the status of provisions through a tube? A partial answer is found in considering if a label makes reality or if reality generates concepts which are labeled. It seems self-evident that the world external to the human mind, extra-mental reality, generates concepts that are labeled.

Knowledge of Human Nature

Human nature is this principle of activity and rest (nature) within a human, bringing life and continuing until death. In this way, human nature is an internal principle.

An Integral Union

As human, we are an integral union between human nature (also called the principle of life, form, or soul) and the materials out of which we are made. A living human has both a material body and this internal principle enlivening the body. This Aristotelian unity of being contrasts with the dualist perspective of Plato and Descartes.

The Dualist Perspective

Dualists consider our immaterial capacities, soul, as dwelling within and communicating with and through the material body, but not united in the way Aristotle calls integral. That is, in such a way that there is not a living biological human without the soul. For the dualist, one could have human biological existence and later the infusion of a human soul completing human nature, and the soul could have left the body behind in conditions like Persistent Vegetative State.

An Immaterial Source

Humans can be seen as an exception to the directive activity of nature giving rise to existence. Natural procreation [parental intercourse] clearly provides for the existence of the body through the unique new DNA at conception, but humans have an immaterial capacity in conceptual thought witnessing the presence of an immaterial soul. In this classical understanding, the immaterial concepts are a higher order of existence than the material body because concepts continue across place and time. The number "2" or the concept of larger or love remains when those thinking about them have long been gone. Considering the long-held position that the lesser cannot produce the greater, we cannot hold that material being gives existence to immaterial being, or the lesser can produce the greater. But, if the immaterial cannot come from the material, an immaterial source is required to give rise to the human soul which has immaterial capacities.

Knowing what can be Known in Nature

What can be known? How is knowledge of nature possible? And, what is it about existent items that make it possible for humans to know them? These are important philosophical questions. That is, of course, if it is possible to know. For the purposes of our discussion we will suppose that the world is intelligible and can be known. However, this question of the skeptic, whether or not we really know the world as it is, always lurks in the background.

It is Possible to Know

As intelligent beings, it is possible to know if we have our clothes on, and to make distinctions like mine and yours. This is common sense support that we can know. Even the skeptic looks both ways before crossing the street. They assume one would know if a car was coming. The response comes back, but one is not safely across the street until he or she reaches the other side and this is so, but does not negate that we looked assuming the capacity to know. Another response is that this is a trivial example. I'm not so sure it is. Knowing involves both experience, logical reasoning from that experience, and past experiences to support our ideas. For example: when looking for traffic, I see no car, and hear no car, so there is probably no car.

Knowing Invisible Capillaries

The 17th Century philosopher Renee Descartes in his treatise, *Discourse on Method*,[27] describes William Harvey's experiments on animals that showed blood circulates and, thus, there must be invisible capillaries. This was prior to microscopic visualization. He showed the

---

[27] Rene' Descartes, *Discourse on Method and Meditations on First Philosophy*. Translated by Donald A. Cress. Indianapolis: Hackett Publishing Co., 1980, part Five, pp.25-28.

heart is a pump and there is a limited volume of blood. With a pump and a limited volume, blood had to flow in a closed system, the fluid moving out from the heart must return to the heart to be used again. In order for blood to return to the heart there must be small pathways in our extremities where the blood changes from moving away to returning back to the heart.

Knowing Nature

When we have knowledge, we could say it is an item's nature that is known, and this is accurate for some things. But, if this were the whole story, it seems we could not know artificial things. So, we have to look further than an item's nature for an answer to what is known in something that is known.

Knowing Number

When we consider the world as a whole, we notice that nature is in a constant state of change or becoming, but this is not true of all that exists. Numbers and geometrical figures, when separated from material things are outside of change. Two is two no matter what "two" describes; two trees or two cats or two clouds. Number does not change. While these trees, cats and clouds are seen as two of each, the two can be separated from the materials of these existent items and added together to make six. In this separated state, number can be used for many calculations providing certain, secure results. Additionally, a number, like two or five, has been two or five from the beginning of time. The same can be said of geometrical figures like the circle or square.

Knowing Statistically

Humans, because of free will, cannot be depended on to act in a given way. Nonetheless, when behaviors are measured the numerical values can be submitted to statistical analysis that can lead to seemingly more secure results. Mathematical developments have enabled increased certitude but cannot overcome the unpredictable human freedom and the indefinite results of future looking studies. Nature only acts generally and for the most part[28] and, yet the circle is always a circle, a line every point equidistant from the center. This variance between mathematics and nature and especially statistics and human functioning means research results

---

[28] Wallace, pp. 19-21.

must be carefully evaluated within the human setting. One cannot assume the study results apply. There are too many variables. One has a responsibility to only tentatively and carefully apply results until one sees a match between the present situation and the circumstances of the research.

Knowing is Having Universals in the Mind

A new piece of information is added to our discussion of knowledge, when we consider that in knowing something the item comes to be in the mind of the knower in a way comparable to its own existence and according to the capacities of the knower. Since number and figure have immaterial existence they are in the mind of the knower in an immaterial way. Items in the world can be known to change but what is known is separated from the change outside of the mind, similar to the way two was separated from two trees, or two cats, or two clouds. Nature is experienced in all of its particularity or individuality but it is known as the intellect grasps the stable separable immaterial content, like tall or brown or tree.

Contemporary Aristotelian Philosopher, Wallace, would say knowledge is of universals rather than particulars.[29] Experiencing particular trees allows us to grasp the universal concept tree. What is known are the universal aspects of the experienced particular? Knowledge is concerned with stable, intelligible content. It seems these objects of knowledge in the mind are more like mathematicals than changeable particular objects in the world. That which is known is the same intelligible component that forms existing substances, the formal of the matter/form unity. If we find the stability within the changes in the world outside of the mind, we will find the stability which constitutes what is known when something is known.

Demonstration on the Assumption of the End

Because nature acts generally and for the most part, predictability is limited. Usually secure knowledge exists only after something has happened. If one has decreased cardiac output, one must balance activity and rest, fluid intake, and sodium intake in order for the heart to keep up with demand and remain compensated, which is having a balance between demand and capacity. Still one can do all these things and decompensate and have edema of the feet (right sided) or in the lungs (left sided). But, if

---

[29] Wallace, pp. 327-332.

one is compensated with demands on the heart within the capacities of the heart, they have done all of these things. This can be formulated as a proof, on the assumption of the end. If one is in cardiac compensation, then he or she has balanced activity and rest, fluid and sodium intake. It can be asserted, the patient is in a state of compensation.

Theodoric of Freiberg (1250-1310) doing research on the rainbow showed that while one cannot ever be sure when there will be a rainbow, without a doubt, if there is a rainbow the required conditions were met, sun and rain and observer at the correct angle to the sun.[30]

Stability Within Change

How do we explain stability within all of the change that we observe and experience? The need to explain both stability and change led Aristotle's famous teacher, Plato, to assert the existence of The **Forms**.[31]

Platonic Forms

These Forms (notice the capitalization) are Eternal Perfections outside the world of change, they contain no matter. In Plato's view participation in The Forms makes every item be what it is, including even non-material things like transcendentals, Unity, Beauty, Truth, and Goodness. For Plato, this earth is like ever-changing sights and sounds about which we only have imaginary explanations. Study and careful science provide generalizations about nature that can be believed, like Harvey's work on the capillaries or Theodoric of Freiburg on the rainbow, but knowledge, what truly is the case, is found only in knowing these unchanging Ideas, the Forms. By participation in The Forms through education, the mind is drawn toward these more stable truths in the world of the intellect. Within this Platonic view, knowledge requires mathematical reasoning and insight into The Forms. The stability of mathematics and objects of thought are intermediate between the unstable world of change and the permanence of the world of The Forms.

Aristotelian Forms

Aristotle explained nature and knowledge of nature without these

---

[30] Aristotle, *Physics*, Bk. II.

[31] Plato, *Republic,* Book Seven. You may want to review "the allegory of the cave" at the beginning of the Seventh Book of the Republic (514a-516b).

other-worldly Eternal Forms. He considered The Forms and the conception of participation as multiplying things to be explained. Aristotle starts his explanation of change by describing the composition of things we experience.[32] Whether natural or artificial, these things that change are **substances**. Each stone is a substance. Flowers, trees, birds, even humans are substances. A substance is an integral union of matter and form. Saying **integral union** means that when we think about them we can separate them but in the actual existing substance they cannot be separate. Thus, when the chemist detects the yellow band of light in the spectrum of sulfur, the element can be positively identified as sulfur. When the student of embryology identifies living tissues as making dog DNA or human DNA, a dog embryo or a human embryo is being observed. **Matter** is that 'out of which' something is made, for example, the carbon, nitrogen, hydrogen, chlorophyll and the other molecules that go into making a crystal, a cat, a tree, or a rose bush. Materials are uniquely patterned under the direction of **form** (notice Aristotle's form is not capitalized). Form is that which makes a thing 'be what it is.' Aristotle would say that at first matter had the **potential** to be all things; quantities of this first or **primary matter** 'take on' form to actually become kinds of elements or kinds of things. This is not in the same way boats take on water. The single marks around 'take on' indicate that the phrase is being used in a unique sense. There is an extent to which these words cannot express what is meant, but matter never is found without form (without being some kind of thing). Initially, matter is potential to receiving all forms, and then it is potential to what the current matter-form unity can become. You may be thinking form sounds a lot like nature discussed above, and so it is for the natural substance.

Matter, either primary or determined, is actualized by form to become all that exists in the world, natural and artificial. As discussed earlier, change natural to a thing comes from within. Form is this internal change agent. A thing's form makes it a particular kind of being. Using our earlier example of a desk, the natural form of the oak or maple tree prepared the wood. Imposition of the artificial form transformed the wood into a desk.

Living Substance is the Integral Unity of Matter Energized by Form

For the living, the natural form is the source of vital activities characteristic of the kind of being it is. We can now say a living substance

---

[32] Wallace, p. 132.

is the integral unity of matter energized by form. Although it is possible to identify two aspects of substance, matter and form, this is not a dualism. The notion of integral unity is critical and captures the distinction between Aristotle and the dualists: Plato and Descartes. In the *Physics,* at 193b3, Aristotle reaffirms the unity of matter and form in natural things by reminding us that matter and form are "not separable except in statement," which we can take to mean in thought and speech.

Matter provides a unique particular physical reality. Matter is the principle that sets apart individuals, the **principle of individuation**. Form is the **principle of stability**, that which is shared by all things specified as the same kind. **Substantial form** is stabilizing, unifying and specifying. The forest is full of individual Redwood trees, all united as Redwood trees by the substantial form that makes them all be what they are by giving rise to the unique attributes of the Redwood. Each item is one instance of the form that is shared with all others of the same kind. And yet, in their individuality they are all different. A shared substantial form with individual material expressions of this form allows for both stability and change. As was said, the intellect grasps form as a concept which we can label and generalize universally to all individual things of the same kind. This capacity to grasp and label concepts gives rise to speech.

The Known

At this important juncture, we see that it is form, natural or artificial, that is grasped by the intellect, identified, labeled and used in speech. Stimuli received by all of the senses are transmitted through inner senses to the intellect. The intellect actively abstracts universal notes as concepts to be labeled by words and applied universally to all items of the same kind. The words used depend on one's language. Specific terms are applied to concepts in the mind. With these concepts expressed in sentences, assertions can be made about the world. Propositions are sentences that assert a predicate belongs to the subject, for instance, "That tree has apples." This assertion can be tested to see if the intellectual grasp of the world corresponds to the factual existence or the way things are. In a common-sense way, we look to see if there are apples growing on the tree. Or, scientifically, through careful reasoning from true premises one can come to new knowledge. The reasoning of Harvey, referred to earlier, proving the existence of pathways to complete the circulatory path from the heart back to the heart was considered as secure as mathematical reasoning by Descartes.[33] These capillaries were available to reason long before their visualization with the microscope. You may think capillaries are so obvious that their proof is trivial, but circulation had been a mystery and discovery of the circulatory path was very significant to seventeenth century health care and likely led the way to I.V. therapy in the modern age.

Conclusion

Form, whether natural or artificial, makes possible knowledge of the world through an intellectual grasp of concepts and the human capacity to reason. For Aristotle, this form exists within all existants, as well as being concepts within the mind of the knower. Once concepts, separated from matter, are grasped, we put words to them and use them to label all other items of the same kind. In this way, assertive sentences are used as premises to support conclusions about our world. Formal logic provides for assessing arguments to support the validity of the line of reasoning. Valid reasoning and true premises allow for secure growth of knowledge.

---

[33] See. n.27.

Conversation Starters:

1. Discuss the following with two or three classmates: Does Aristotle or Plato's position on the nature of existence seem stronger to you? Prepare a group response in the form of an argument with assertive premises concluding to the chosen position.

   a. Plato holds that individuals are a particular kind with particular attributes because they share, or participate, in Forms of that kind. There are eternal Forms for each major kind of being and attributes, like colors, and the transcendentals like Beauty, Truth, Goodness and Unity (evil is a lack of Goodness and illness is a lack of Unity). Human souls dwell in the realm of Forms until they come to reside in a body on earth. Humans return to the perfect realm of forms by seeking knowledge and virtue.

   b. Aristotle holds that individuals are substances that are integral unities of matter and form. These individuals are what they are and have their attributes from their internal principle of activity and rest, which is their form or soul, also called essence or nature. Attributes are essential to the kind they are or accidental and do not impact the kind they are. Virtue is a habit of acting well and evil is chosen. Beauty, truth, goodness and unity are important as attributes that cross space and time, but are not something separate from items that express them and the humans that grasp them as transcendent concepts. Nonetheless, chosen evil is still a lack of goodness or wisdom, and illness is a lack of unity and proper function.

2. With a classmate, read and discuss your ideas on the following:
   a. "The Allegory of the Cave" at the beginning of the Seventh Book of Plato's Republic (514a-516b).
   b. Section b on Aristotle in item 2 above.

   Using one of these, draw or write a description of health care services thinking on stability, progress, and leadership. You will share some insights from your group work with the class.

Reflection Submissions:

1. From reading Plato and Aristotle, including the Conversation Starter Chapter 3-1, do humans have souls dwelling in bodies or souls united to the materials of the body. Support your answer.

2. Animals like birds and mammals have to shelter from the heat, cold, rain and sun. Bird nests are said to be by nature because each kind of bird builds the same nest as all other birds of that kind.

Considering human shelters, what about the shelter is natural and what is artificial. Be sure to begin with definitions of natural and artificial.

Outline for Chapter 3: Foundations of Knowing Nature and Human Nature
   A.   Philosophy of Nature
       1. Seeking a stable source of moral guidance
       2. Other sources of moral guidance
       3. Moving to the knowledge of human nature
   B. Forms of Logical Reasoning
       1. Valid logical forms of reasoning
           a. Modus Ponens
           b. Modus Tollens
       2. Invalid logical forms of reasoning
           a. The fallacy of denying the antecedent
           b. The fallacy of affirming the consequent
   C. Knowledge of Nature
       1. Nature as the world
       2. Nature as an internal principle
   D. Natural and Artificial
   E. Knowledge of Human Nature
       1. An integral union
       2. The dualist perspective
       3. An immaterial source
   F. Knowing What can be Known in Nature
       1. It is possible to know
           a. Invisible capillaries
           b. Nature
           c. Number
           d. Statistics
       2. Knowing is having universals in the mind
       3. Demonstrations on the assumption of the end
   G. Stability within Change
       1. Platonic forms
       2. Aristotelian forms
       3. Living substances is the integral unity of matter energized by form
   H. The Known
   I. Conclusion

Terminology for Chapter 3
Antecedent
Consequent
Modus Ponens
Modus Tollens
Fallacies
Nature
Artifact
Artificial
Natural
Persistent Vegetative State (PVS)
Substance
Integral union
Matter
Form
Primary matter
Principle of individuation
Principle of stability
Substantial form

CHAPTER 4

HUMANS AS PERSONS IN COMMUNITY

Objectives

After studying this chapter, you will be able to:

1. Compare animal and human life identifying the unique capacities of humans.
2. Describe humanity in terms of essential and accidental properties attributed to humans.
3. Describe being human in terms of the substantial, relational and transcendent synthesis of Norris Clarke.
4. Recognize the difference in community experienced by Karen Ann Quinlan and Terry Schiavo.
5. Consider lessons from the health-care community in its early adjustment to comatose patients.
6. Describe the framework and theory of Imogene King in its contribution to making philosophy accessible to health-care practitioners.

Properties of Human Nature

Within Chapter Three we learned substantial form (nature) is the internal energizing principle of the matter-form unity of a living substance. Substantial form makes an individual the kind of being that it is. In this development, this energizing principle gives rise to the primary properties essential to the kind of being that is developing. These properties and capacities allow us to recognize something as what it is. For example, squirrels are of a particular shape and size, live in trees, and have the habit of storing food for the winter. We can argue whether squirrels are black, gray, gray and white or brown or we can even agree that they are all of these colors, but we recognize the squirrel as squirrel because of its natural substantial form. Characteristic behaviors assist us in this identification but, identification of the thing being discussed is necessary in order to dispute about secondary properties, like fur color. Certain attributes or properties generate directly from the nature of the being, from its substantial form, and are thus said to be **essential** to what the individual is. Other attributes, like color, are specific to particular individuals and are thus said to be **accidental**, or secondary (not essential to the kind of being). These secondary attributes are actualized by accidental form. Even though it is genetically determined whether a particular squirrel will be black or gray, color is secondary to its being a squirrel. On the other hand, storing food for the winter is essential; it is within the squirrel's nature to do so.

In this understanding, substance has a principle of individuation and change (matter) and a principle of universality and stability (form). What is known within all of the change we experience in our world are essential and accidental forms, which come to be universal concepts in the mind. These concepts are immaterial because they leave matter behind and are more stable than the world outside of the mind. For example, the tree in the yard comes to be in the human inner senses (aspects of the brain) as an image, a replica of the tree experienced. The intellect abstracts intelligible notes forming concepts in the mind. Essential form is a thing's nature, the actualizing principle that makes each kind be what it is. Accidental or secondary form provides for unique aspects of individuals. Each member of a kind of being is identifiable by its expression of its essential and accidental forms.

One of the goals of this chapter is to capture the essential form of being human. We ask, "What attributes are essential and define being human?" The most obvious answer is the intellectual capacities, as they are uniquely human; these include reasoning with immaterial concepts and freedom of choice based on knowledge. We will then discuss Norris Clarke's classic and contemporary descriptions of being human as matter-form unities, substantial beings, whose relationality and self-transcendence takes one into communion with others. Review of the landmark cases of Karen Ann Quinlan and Terry Schiavo reveal how the comatose individual is still a person in community. Karen Ann was the first comatose person placed on a ventilator who did not awaken or die within a short period of time. Reading experiences of her sister and mother highlight how the health-care community had to learn to be caregivers in this new situation. Finally, we will consider how Imogene King's framework and theory apply essential human properties in clinical practice. According to King, respect for an individual's capacities of reason and freedom (self-determination) enhances health through mutual goal setting.[34]

---

[34] King, I. M. (1981). *A theory for nursing: Systems, concepts, processes*. New

Nature was previously defined as an internal principle of activity and rest. This inner dimension that gives existence and guides development of an individual as a particular natural kind is not visible in itself. This energizing nature is internal and unobservable except in union with matter. We become aware of its presence through its material and formal effects, as when an acorn sprouts and sets its roots deep into the ground and the little stem moves upward toward the sky. We experience the effects of natural form in every natural substance. These characteristic effects allow us to identify individuals of a particular kind as members of that kind. It was noted in Chapter Three, that human nature, the soul, was immaterial because the soul is capable of immaterial thought. This immateriality of the soul led to the conclusion that there must be an immaterial source for this unique immaterial human soul.

Humans as the Knowing Subject (Knower)

Humans are not the only beings in the world that come to know. Animals and humans both have sensory knowledge. This knowledge is closely related to experience of the external world. It requires sensory abilities provided by at least some outer senses. The capacities of the nervous system called inner senses coordinate the sensations and through memory and imagination fill in details not directly available within a particular experience.

The Senses

For humans, the outer senses are vision, hearing, smell, taste, and touch. The inner senses are a category not usually spoken of in this way outside of classical philosophy. They were identified and used by Aristotle, Aquinas, and Wallace. However, parallels to this classical explanation can be found in contemporary psychology of perception.[35] The inner senses are the central or coordinating sense, memory, and imagination that provide a unified image or perception from the received sensations. Because of human cognition, the fourth inner sense is called **cogitative**; in animals it is called the **estimative** sense, as it provides an immediate estimate of desirable or harmful. In either case, it is an immediate estimate whether the encountered situation is safe. It is especially important in its role in avoiding harm.

York: Wiley.
[35] http://allpsych.com/psychology101/perception.html.

The cogitative capacity can be seen in the following scenario. One evening, leaving a pharmacy at closing time, you forgot to pull the keys to have them in your hand. As you walked to your car, the hairs on the back of your neck begin to stand up and you feel an inner tension. You process what you ought to do. You realize you did not have keys in hand, but you knew to not to start looking them. You decide to turn suddenly and as fast as you can, return to the store. As you make a sharp U-turn, you push past three large men. In this event, we can say physical intuitions interfaced with reason. This is cogitative, the immediate perception of harm.

Human Intellectual Capacities

Human knowing[36] moves beyond the problem-solving capacities of animals because of the ability to think about and to reason from immaterial concepts organized into sentences and propositions used as premises and conclusions of arguments. There are two **modally distinct** capacities of the intellect. The phrase 'modally distinct' means that we can separate them when we think about them, but they are not actually separate. These capacities are **intellect** itself and the appetite of the intellect, the **will**. The intellect abstracts concepts and organizes them into statements (propositions) that can then be judged to be true or false. A statement is true to the extent it agrees with the way the world is. The statement may be completely true, partially true, or completely in error and thus, false. With true premises, the intellect can reason to confirm ideas as new knowledge. Concept formation, judgment, and reasoning are the three acts of the mind. These were used in the previous example of the perception of danger where one's judgment of danger was probably real given the lateness of the hour and the location. We reasoned to a safe action and in doing this action, confirmed the initial assessment by running into the men that were following. Reasoning to new knowledge was present in Harvey's discovery of the distant pathways in the extremities between arterioles and venules.[37] This required that he develop new ideas, conduct experiments to prove hypotheses, and to reason to the existence of distal pathways now named the capillaries.

---

[36] This work is summarized from Wallace, *Modeling,* pp. 114-131.
[37] Translated D. A. Cress, Rene Descartes, *Discourse on Method*, Part Five, 47-55. Indianapolis, Hackett, 1980.

The Will as Appetite

The will, the appetite of the intellect, moves one to action or prevents one through a negative response according to what is known. When something is known it can be desired or avoided. Since desire energizes and moves to action, limiting knowledge limits choices. Human freedom requires knowledge of options and the physical and emotional freedom to act on the known options. What we call the will may be presented with the most rational or the most desirable option for a number of reasons, but it is within human freedom to choose to act differently.

An Excellent Human Life

Because of the human ability to grasp concepts from the world outside of the mind, it is possible to know what it is to be human as a kind of being in the world. And, what it would be to live an excellent human life, developing the best of human capacities, the virtues. This grasp of human nature or "humanity," said universally, provides principles that explain and prescribe how humans ought to act and to be treated. This knowledge is abstract, that is of humanity, not of Mary, Sue, or John in their circumstances at this time. Knowledge of how humans can live a harmonious productive life is the professional caregiver's interface with virtue, and the moral foundations for ethical decision making.

Respect for Others

For Aristotle (417 a 20.)[38], recognition of the other as one of the human kind makes clear potentials and calls us to respect the other as human with capacity for knowledge and personal choice based on knowledge. Aristotle may think this recognition of human dignity ought to guarantee respect and protections. Nonetheless, through great periods of history, even now individuals and ethnic groups have been treated as less than human and people are murdered every day. These individuals have not been respected as the unique, valuable human persons they are.

---

[38] *On the Soul*, Translated J.A. Smith, in *The Basic Works of Aristotle,* Richard McKeon, editor. New York: Random House, Inc. 1941. pp. 535-603.

Characteristic Capacities of Beings

On the most elementary level, in order to know, one has to be alive and capable of sensitive life as well as rational life. For a fuller understanding of human life as compared to other living beings, we will use Wallace's work to look briefly at the characteristic capacities of each level of being in the world, even including the non-living inorganic aspects of nature, like minerals, stones. Minimal capacities of living things are nutrition, growth and development, reproduction, and homeostasis (the ability to adapt to the environment). Except for borderline existences like viruses, living organisms are composed of cells and cellular constituents, like mitochondria and nucleic acids which are biochemical, composed of ions, nitrogen, carbon and oxygen. All chemicals, organic and inorganic, respond to an internal structure that makes them be what they are. Chemicals and the non-living material substances of earth are characterized by four powers: the strong forces, weak forces, electromagnetic forces, and gravity. These capacities of natural elements enter in to the capacities of all living things.

Animals are sensitive beings in our world. They are said to be sensitive because they have capacities of sensation, as well as emotional or sensitive responses to the environment. In addition to the above eight capacities that allow for living plants, animals have outer senses and the inner senses already discussed that allow for perception and the problem-solving capacities of sensory knowledge. Animals also have desires or appetites and the ability to move to fulfill these desires or to act on responses to escape harm. Animal life has twelve capacities: the four inorganic powers, the four vegetative powers and the four powers required for sensitive life; outer senses, inner senses, emotion/appetite and motor capacities.

Humans are the Rational Animals

As Aristotle so clearly noted, in his discussion *On the Soul*,[39] humans are the rational animals. As animals we share with all animals the characteristic of sensitive life. But as human, we must add the rational capacities of intellect and will. The intellectual ability to abstract immaterial concepts from perceptions gained through experience provides the most characteristic, essential capacity of human life. This highest human capacity is respected when one provides knowledge needed for personal choice. Preservation of life may be the priority in emergency

---

[39] Ibid.

settings, then pain and symptom control. Health education becomes the priority once the patient is stabilized. Following the pattern of the inorganic, vegetative, sensitive and then rational capacities, priorities may be identified to preserve life, stabilize functioning of systems, processing of behavioral responses, and then health education and mutual goal setting.[40] To be human is to belong to the kind of beings who have the potential to know the world on an immaterial universal level. Joined with this essential property of knowledge is the other essential capacity for freedom of choice. Because humans can anticipate the future, we laugh when startled that the expected did not happen or the unexpected happens. Since the ability to laugh follows immediately on essential capacities, to laugh is said to be an essential human property. Height, weight, hair color, skin tone, or being artistically inclined are accidental properties characterizing individuals.

Aquinas on Immateriality[41]

Aquinas argues that because of our immaterial capacities, humans have an immaterial soul; a principle of life that cannot come from the materials out of which we are made. Evidence of this immateriality is the minds ability to grasp immaterial enduring mathematical figures and formula as well as universal concepts, especially ideas of truth, beauty, goodness, and love. He would argue that at death the body deteriorates but the soul continues. Matter decays, not form. As the human soul, this immaterial form with immaterial capacities has no parts so cannot fall apart.

Health and Virtue

As matter-form unities, humans are dynamic living beings. When we have well-functioning bodily capacities, we are said to be healthy. **Health** is a state of excellence with the proper functioning of the inorganic, vegetative, sensitive and intellectual capacities. **Virtue** is to the soul as health is to the body. Just as we must make healthy choices to stay healthy,

---

[40] The phrase "mutual goal setting" is found in the theory of Imogene King, who grounded her nursing theory on humans as unique in capacities of knowledge and freedom of choice. Whelton, B. J. B."The Nursing Act is an Excellent Human Act: A Philosophical Analysis Derived from Classical Philosophy and the Conceptual Framework and Theory of Imogene King," Chapter Two, *Middle Range Theory Development Using King's Conceptual System,* Christina Leibold Sieloff and Maureen Fry (editors), New York: Springer Publishing Company, 2007, pp. 12-28.
[41] Gleaned from Summa Theologicae Questions 84 and 85.

we need to make virtuous choices to be a well-functioning, virtuous person. Aristotle writes, "It must then be remarked that every virtue or excellence (1) renders good the thing itself of which it is the excellence, and (2) causes it to perform its function well."[42]To a great extent the virtues prepare us to interact with other persons in the environment.

Social Beings

As relational social beings we participate in the world connecting ourselves to others in families, friendships, and communities. We gain our self-awareness from the way we are treated by significant persons in our interpersonal environment. We come to know ourselves as capable, loving, and fun to be with because other people have treated us as capable, loving and fun.

Those humans unable to achieve self-awareness (self-consciousness) still communicate themselves to others in their environment through physiological and emotional processes. Actually, there is a sense in which all beings communicate themselves to the world. They communicate themselves as stone, plant, animals or humans. This self-communication is a part of existence. With humans this self-communication and receptivity to the communication of others overflows (transcends) the self, creating relationships with others. This overflowing relationality weaves relationships into community. Clarke writes that our substantial being, "tends naturally towards modes of being-together…Being and community are inseparable.[43]

Much human despair seems to emerge from the inability to build this community. What Clarke is saying seems to be more of an ideal than a reality but we can use the idea that we are and need to be beings in relationship to grasp the importance of building community for individuals in long term care settings.

Self-consciousness

Self-consciousness is a term often used in conjunction with humans. Sometimes referred to as self-awareness, in phenomenological language it can be seen as self-presence. This self-presence is an objective distance providing awareness of one's self both as present to one's self and others and as the source of one's actions. This self-awareness enables the person

---

[42] Aristotle, *Ethics*, Book II, Ch. 6, p. 41. See also, Chapter Three, n.20 .
[43] W. Norris Clarke, *Person and Being.* Marquette University Press, 1993, fourth printing, 1998. pp. 13-15.

to meaningfully say "I." The human journey is a social one. Humans are social in nature, we are from the beginning a self in relationship. Our receptivity to others leads to loving self-transcendence, which is an overflowing of self towards others.[44]

Sleeping Beauty

Consider for a moment the childhood tale of Sleeping Beauty. The beautiful princess is asleep from a supernatural spell. It's been about a hundred years later when a handsome prince stumbles upon the castle tangled with vines. Curiosity brings him to clear a path and enter the castle. He is mysteriously drawn to find the sleeping girl, who has not aged while she was sleeping unaware of her surroundings. Falling in love with her beauty and innocence he kisses her. She immediately awakens as does everything in her environment.

The story of Sleeping Beauty can be seen as a coming of age tale, or of the deeper reality that we cannot awaken to who we are as a person and to the actual exercise of our self-determining capacities until someone else appreciates and nourishes our being. In the language of phenomenology, "Unless someone else treats me as a "thou" I can never wake up to myself as an "I," as a person."[45] Reflecting on who I am as human, Clarke would say "I distinguish myself from the subhuman world around me by responding to it, by interacting with it and discovering that it is not like me, neither articulate, nor self-conscious, not free, as I am."[46] In community, we come to see who we are as human persons, to acknowledge our own being, to develop our capacities to communicate, and to transcend ourselves in communion as our natural fulfillment.

Lessons from Quinlan and Schiavo

April 15, 1975, a beautiful young lady was at a party, she may have taken a tranquilizer. One can imagine she may have been anxious and a friend offered her a valium before the party so she could enjoy herself. During the party she had a few drinks. Later that evening she was found nonresponsive and she was not breathing. The person who found her started CPR (cardiopulmonary resuscitation). The ambulance arrived and the responders were able to restore oxygenation of her body through CPR.

---

[44] Clark .p. 42.
[45] Clarke, p.45.
[46] Clark, p.65.

There may have been a mechanical hand held bag for breathing called an Ambu ventilator. When the chemicals ought to have been worn off, she still did not breathe on her own. She had been without oxygen for too long.

Approximately, 1964, Byrd Ventilators were introduced into the Intensive Care Unit. Over the next several years the equipment became more and more sophisticated and technologically responsive. The specialization of Respiratory Therapist emerged to answer the need for health-care professionals with advanced knowledge and training in the use of this specialized technology.

Ventilators are wonderful but created dilemmas. They can breathe for an injured person until spontaneous breathing is restored by reduction in brain swelling. They may bypass the oral cavity to increase the air available to the lower smaller air passageways (alveoli) where carbon dioxide and oxygen transfer (respiration) occurs. With a crushed chest, the ventilator could maintain sufficient lung expansion for ventilation and to prevent life threatening pneumonia. Their introduction was an exciting improvement in health care. Nonetheless, ventilators also brought with them some of the most difficult situations. Severely brain injured persons could now be kept alive for prolonged periods by artificial ventilation. Persons, who would have quietly and naturally died, now would not die as long as they were ventilated and their heart did not stop. Guidelines were needed in their use and in their discontinued use.

These momentous decisions were addressed in the battle to have Karen Ann Quinlan's ventilator removed. Karen was found unresponsive and not breathing after a party. Ventilators seemed perfect for making available oxygenated air during times of drug induced apnea. When the effect of chemicals wore off, the ventilator would be removed. In 1975, no one had yet removed a ventilator when they believed the patient would not breathe on their own. Physicians and other caregivers feared they would be committing murder. Even when the court order said they would not be tried for homicide they were afraid to remove the equipment, probably based on moral accountability. The removal of the ventilator seemed like putting a pillow over Karen's face so she could not breathe. Yet, there is a critical difference because air is available if the patient's body responds by breathing.

When it became clear that Karen would not awaken, the physicians and nurses distanced themselves. This distance is starkly presented in the rudeness of a nurse captured in the memory of Karen's sister and quoted in a memoir written thirty years later by Karen's mother, Julia Duane

Quinlan.[47] Quinlan retells Mary Ellen's experience when she went to see her sister for the first time in the ICU. This is a long quotation but so clearly expresses the disappointment that Karen did not recover and the nurse's apparent indifference. In the early days of technological success, health care professionals had little experience or reserve to cope with failure and the distress of families. In the memoir written thirty years later, Julia Quinlan writes of Mary Ellen's experience:

> The first time I went to see Karen in Newton Memorial Hospital, the intensive care unit nurse questioned me intensely.
> "Only close relatives are permitted in. How do I know you're related?" Finally, unsatisfied but realizing I wasn't going to leave, she said, "Go ahead. If you like to see people like that."
> Not especially liking to see people like that, particularly the person I most relied on to live forever, I went in anyway.
> Much later thinking about my first look at Karen in the hospital bed, her blood from the emergency trachea just done splattered on the white sheets and pillow, I understood the attitude of the ICU nurse. Karen was one of their failures, in a world where technology replaces comfort and caring, where organs are transplanted from the dead so the living can cling to life and the business of medicine is managed by strangers. Karen was beyond help. Somebody no one wanted to look at.
> Four months after my first look the world looked. A long terrifying look at the value of life and its qualities. The void between caring and curing (sic). The extraordinary distance medical technology will go before admitting failure. As the lines were drawn between machines and medicine, law and justice, life and death, the world couldn't look away. For the next ten years, we couldn't either.[48] (The expression and style of the author preserved).

This is not included to criticize the courageous staff that cared for Karen but for you to be aware of how technology changed the face of care and with these changes came new challenges. There will be new challenges encountered in your practice. In all of these changes it is now expected that health care practitioners will be aware of the impact of their words and sensitive to the emotional needs of family members.

Late in May, 1975, Julia Quinlan faced the reality that Karen was not going to improve. She expresses changes in approach that are today's standards of care, but were not yet. Again, I feel it is worth providing a significant portion of her thinking to assist awareness as we strive to provide care in these difficult situations.

---

[47] *My Joy, My Sorrow*, Cincinnati, Ohio: St Anthony Messenger Press, 2005, p.39.
[48] Mary Ellen Quinlan-Forzano, 2004. In Quinlan. p.39.

I began to question myself as to why she was still on the machines. I felt that now the emphasis should be on caring for Karen in a more compassionate way. In a way that would be good for Karen, not just those who did not want to let her go. Loving support was more important and humane than life-preserving, death-defying procedures. I could not share my feelings with my family; they were not prepared to listen to any hints that she might not recover.[49]

When the Quinlans went to court in November 1975 to seek authority to have her ventilator removed, their goal was not her death. They wanted the extraordinary treatments stopped. Quinlan writes, "We wanted our daughter returned to a natural state without the maze of technology. We wanted our daughter to be able to die a natural and peaceful death." For this person who became the first icon of the "right to die" the goal was not death but the removal of extraordinary means. Her family did not want her to die; they wanted to be able to be close to her without the distancing equipment. Initially the court ruled that Mr. Quinlan was too deeply involved with loving his daughter to make this decision. Six months later, March 31, 1976, a year after the fateful event, the New Jersey Supreme Court in a right to privacy decision ruled that this very involvement was what is required for such a decision.

In all of these events Karen Ann was clearly within the arms of her family, community, and then the world. Her family did not want her to die; they wanted her to be in a natural state receiving care that would make her life as comfortable as possible. May 22nd the weaning process was over and she was still breathing. When they went home, the family prayed that she would still be there for them the next day.[50] Having been successfully weaned from the ventilator, Karen was transferred from the hospital to a long-term care facility. From the perspective of community and persons in community, let us note that every day from the day of her injury Karen's mother and father went to visit her. They told her about the happenings of their day, shared music and prayers with her. She was very much still a part of their family, and would be for another ten years.

When Karen Ann was first resuscitated the need was to restore oxygenation of the tissues, especially the brain. This was done mechanically. At the edge of life and death, biochemical balance is critical to maintain the matter form unity of the living substantial being. Admitted to the Intensive Care Unit issues of fluid balance and nutrition, skin integrity, and sensations emerge. As comatose Karen Ann could only communicate biochemical and

---

[49] Quinlan, p.41-2.
[50] Quinlan, p.54.

behavioral responses, like a fever or redness and swelling of pressure. Her respiratory responses were not synchronized with the ventilator, her body fought the ventilator. Her mother relates this as "watching her struggle to release herself from the machine."[51] The ability of health professionals to resolve this stress came years later with medications to assist the ventilator patient to accept assistance. And ethically, after years of deliberation addressing quality of life, when life ends, and the distinctions between killing and letting die health-care professionals have many more resources with which to assist patients and families.

Although not known in 1975, we know today that someone in deep coma may still hear. Karen Ann's parents provided audio and tactile stimulation unsure what she could hear, but she did startle with sudden sounds. Maintained as a substantial being self-communication and existence was on a non-rational level.

The family system was threatened by her injury and unresponsiveness. By daily visits Karen remained related as a member of the family. When she entered the emergency room and then ICU, she entered into health-care communities. The health professionals were uncertain how to relate to this unresponsive young lady and her dedicated family. An outrageous exchange occurred at the hospital after the court order and while the Quinlans were finding a nursing center for her. Julia Quinlan writes, "Because of the New Jersey Supreme Court decision and the hospital's reluctance to abide by the decision, we had little contact with her doctor. He avoided us whenever possible until one day when he approached Joe and me in the hallway. He asked that we stop our daily visits, since they were upsetting the nurses."[52] It seems unbelievable that a health-care professional would be so insensitive. I believe this comment reflects the threat and sorrow felt by a community of caregivers prepared to cure but not to see care, just caring for someone and their family as valued professional activity. Today this provision of care when cure is not possible is called palliative care.

"Cure may be futile but care is never futile."[51]

Writing nearly twenty years later the physician-ethicist, Edmund Pellegrino expresses the more contemporary view of professional care in the presence of irreparable injury or terminal illness. He writes,

> "Often, the meaning of the word health, namely 'making whole again', cannot be achieved, but much can still be done to restore harmony or physiological and psychological function. To care, comfort, be present,

---

[51] Quinlan, p.50.
[52] Quinlan, p.63.

help with coping, and to alleviate pain and suffering are healing acts as well as cure. In this sense, healing can occur when the patient is dying even when cure is impossible. Palliative care is a healing act adjusted to the good possible even in the face of the realities of an incurable illness. Cure may be futile but care is never futile."[53]

We earlier read Julia Quinlan express that it was time to discontinue the extraordinary interventions and just take care of Karen as she presented herself, unconscious and totally dependent. This "taking care of" would have been palliative care with the use of ordinary means like food, fluids, and antibiotics.

The layers of communities surrounding Karen Ann had no experience removing lifesaving equipment. They were unable to respond more humanly. They seem to have been trying to protect themselves from the fear of failure and loss, but they had little experience to prepare them for this failure (as they saw it). Sharing this account helps us to anticipate a time when we will confront these issues and to see the critical significance of relationships within a family and health-care community

We have just considered Karen Ann Quinlan, who was part of a close family system within which she had a secure personal identity. Disagreement between this family and the then current standard of health-care practice required a legal decision, one which became a landmark case in allowing removal of the ventilator as an extraordinary intervention at the request of a surrogate decision maker. When the ventilator was removed Quinlan was able to breathe unassisted. Ten years later she died of an infection. During the course of her care she had had antibiotics for infection but at this late period of her life antibiotics were seen as an extraordinary non-obligatory intervention.

Terri Schiavo

In the account of Terri Schiavo, her physical and mental condition, her family, court rulings and finally death were widely publicized. Terri is believed to have suffered severe loss of cerebral function following an electrolyte imbalance that induced a heart attack. Although disputed, she was believed to be in a persistent vegetative state (PVS). She was kept alive for years through the provision of food and fluids. Rather than the ventilator, this case concerned the removal of what had previously been considered ordinary care, food and fluids. This removal was specifically so that Terri might die. The request was made by her surrogate decision

---

[53] E. D. Pellegrino, "The Metamorphosis of Medical Ethics: a 30-year retrospective," *JAMA,* March 3, 1993 (269.9) 1158-1162. (p. 1162).

maker, her husband. To use the word husband entails its legal status, but this man was living with another woman with whom he already had two children. Additionally, when Terri died he would inherit the remainder of her award provided for rehabilitation therapy which was discontinued at his request shortly after the award was made. Some would see this inheritance and living with another woman as disqualifying Michael as surrogate. Living with and having children by another woman seems to make him more akin to an ex-husband than a husband. Ex-husbands are not generally accepted as health-care advocates for the estranged spouse. The right to refuse treatment is a protected legal right, but it requires documentation. Without documentation and without mental capacity a surrogate health care agent is required. Even though the person may have been married only a short time, the spouse is normally the legal surrogate because the incapacitated individual freely chose this person as their life mate; their representative. And, so the Florida court accepted him for making life ending decisions in Terri's care.

In contrast to the Quinlan family, Terri Schiavo's family was divided and filled with conflict. The Schindlers, Terri's parents, pushed for therapy and increasing Terri's capacity at all costs. While her husband seemed to have wanted to save money won for her therapy even if her potential capacities dissipated. He apparently did not see her as having capacity. Her tomb stone tells the story from his perspective. He crafted what it says, "Born December 3, 1963, Departed This Earth, February 25, 1990, At Peace March 31, 2005."[54]

Within her person, Terri was capable of all biological functions. She may also have had some emotional capacity. Interpretations of her cognitive capacities were varied reflecting the values of the one interpreting. Members of euthanasia organizations saw her as being forced to stay alive in a PVS. A neurosurgeon within the Catholic Pro-Life tradition saw her as having minimal cognitive function, but clearly responsive to the environment; a mental state just above PVS.

Right to Refuse Medical Interventions

It had been decided years before with the case of Nancy Cuzan[55] that the mentally impaired retained through written documentation or their

---

[54] http://www.stonescryout.org/archives/2005/06/schiavo_tombsto.html, accessed June 28, 2014.
[55] http://www.casebriefs.com/blog/law/constitutional-law/constitutional-law-keyed-to-stone/implied-fundamental-rights/cruzan-v-director-missouri-department-of-health-2/, accessed June 29, 2014.

surrogate the right to refuse medical interventions. Food and fluids became qualified as medical intervention because gastric tube nutrition is medically prescribed with the tube surgically placed. Whether it is ordinary or extraordinary care became a matter of interpretation and possibly no longer legally relevant if self-determination allows one to refuse any intervention. Moral issues remain around the question of ordinary care being obligatory and a requirement that health care professionals working to heal persons in their care, do not kill. One must decide if removal of nutrition and fluids in the current situation is letting nature take its course and the person dies (letting die), or is this a case of killing the person, setting up an internal environment so that the person will die.

The ultimate and landmark decision for Terri Schiavo was to remove the source of fluids and nutrition that she might die. It seems food and fluids were seen as preventing her death as opposed to bringing nourishment and comfort. Her physiologic and social status was similar to Quinlan but the intent was very different. Quinlan ultimately died of an infection. After ten years of slow decline antibiotics were seen as extraordinary and unnecessary care. Schiavo died of dehydration.

Knowledge and Choice are the Basis of Self-determination

The capacities for reasoning based on conceptual knowledge and choosing among options is the foundation of the important principle of self-determination. **Autonomy** is a respect for these personal choices. Within health care, autonomy is often operative as **informed consent**. Prior to admission to a clinic or hospital, consent to treat is required. Before a procedure informed consent specific to the value and risks of the procedure is required. In order to fulfill this requirement, the patient or health care surrogate (agent) must receive clear and accurate instructions sufficient to decide if the procedure is in the best interest of the patient. The standard of instruction in health care cannot be less than that for making a decision on a sofa or a car, which is, what the reasonable person would need to know. This reasonable-person standard plays an important role in business and health-care ethics as the expected standard of disclosure.

Health care has transitioned from **paternalism,** where patients were told and usually accepted what the physician said was good for them, to **autonomy** where the health care providers accommodate what the patient and/or family want. Nevertheless, it would seem that with the years of education the professional has, one needs to respect their health-care knowledge even while participating in decisions about care. The educator and nursing theorist, Imogene King proposed that mutual goal setting resulting from practitioner and patient/family interactions and transactions, respects both patient and practitioner. This perspective will be further developed shortly.

All Life is Worth Living; Some Interventions are not Worth Having

Thus far, we have developed how humans come to knowledge and how it is possible to have knowledge of humans. This is very important if we are going to have moral principles grounded in human life. The natural/artificial distinction offers some assistance when we consider interventions at the beginning and end of life. That which is natural will work with the patient's life processes, for example intravenous (IV) or nasogastric food and fluids to meet the metabolic demands of multiple wounds or burns. Artificial interventions are imposed on the patient, i.e. mechanical ventilation with pneumonia provides life preserving oxygen while antibiotics reduce the organism's virulence and the need for a mucous producing response. Nonetheless, the patient must be sedated to accept mechanical ventilation and it may be prolonging death when the patient has multisystem failure or irreversible damage from metastatic disease. Even in multisystem failure, for some patients food and fluids may be seen as providing comfort as opposed to prolonging death.

Humans as Substantial, Relational, and Transcendent

In his book, *Person and Being* (1998)[56] the contemporary philosopher, Norris Clarke (1915 – 2008) extended the philosophical understanding that humans are the rational animals to humans are substantial, relational, and transcendent beings who find fulfillment in communion with others, in community through self-possession (having unity and boundaries), self-communication (an attribute of all being to generate phenomena that reveal themselves), and self-transcendence (an over-flowing of the inner-self towards others characteristic of rational being). Individual persons transcend themselves moving toward others with the resultant formation of communities. This capacity for communion is a shared natural human capacity. An individual human (matter/form unity) comes into existence as substantial being, as something-in-itself, with an inner-privacy and the

---

[56] W. Norris Clarke, *Person and Being.* Marquette University Press, 1993, fourth printing, 1998.

potential for self-transcendence and future self-conscious awareness. This new substantial being communicates its presence in utero; at implantation it is self-communicating through biochemistry. The conceptus generates chemicals that interact with the endometrium of the uterine wall and stimulate hormone production declaring its presence and collaborating with the mother's body toward implantation.[57] In this self-announcement, the embryo enters into the environment and into communion with his or her mother; this communion is the new beings first community. Throughout life, according to Clarke, community relationships allow, even encourage, persons to emerge as who they are. Notice the transition from human to person. The ancient philosopher Boethius (ca. 480-524) laid the foundation of a person as "an individual substance of a rational nature." In contrast to slaves, a person "owns" its own act of existence.[58] Clarke extends this, "A personal being is therefore one that is in charge of its own life, a *self-governing being.*"[59] "To be a person is to be intrinsically expansive, ordered toward self-manifestation and self-communication."[60] Thus, humans are a particular kind of being having characteristic behaviors shared with all other humans, as we are all of the same kind. This sameness is our shared nature or essence. Even so, we each have a unique interiority, privacy and an inner self. Philosophically, there is tension between our having this shared universal human nature and each one of us being a unique particular individual.

The previously noted realists' perspectives on substantial being, presented from the work of Wallace, are extended here from views held by Clarke. He contrasts with existentialists, like Sartre, who teaches that we come into existence and then participate in making ourselves and what the world will be, even what it will be to be human in the distant future. There are no stable natures, or kinds of beings in the existentialist perspective. For Sartre, humanity is today the culmination of decisions and activities of

---

[57] From the web site, https://academic.oup.com/humupd/article/13/4/365/2457882
The role of the endometrium and embryo in human implantation
K. Diedrich B.C.J.M. Fauser P. Devroey G. Griesinger on behalf of the Evian Annual Reproduction (EVAR) Workshop Group. *Human Reproduction Update*, Volume 13, Issue 4, 1 July 2007, Pages 365–377,
https://doi.org/10.1093/humupd/dmm011.
For further information on development of the molecular embryo see: Fertilization and molecular embryonic development may be found in the work of Derrick Rancourt at the site "the virtual embryo"
people.ucalgary.ca/~browder/virtualembryo
[58] Clark, p.27.
[59] Clark, p.49.
[60] Clark, p.71.

all who have lived. Future humanity is what we will make it. Another important perspective is that of the phenomenologists like Hegel and Heidegger. In their view, existence is tied to relationships. We are not just characterized by relationships; we exist as the web of our relationships.[61] Clarke wants us to see that we need all three of these perspectives to grasp what it is to be human. We are substantial matter/form unities who travel through time creating our world and building relational communities. According to Clarke, substantiality (being in-itself) and relationality (being towards-others) come into existence together and are inseparable modes of reality.[62]

Summarizing Clarke, we are Aristotelian *substances* with phenomenal *relationality*. We freely made our history and make our future. Substantiality and relationality are equally first and are inseparable modes of reality. **Substantiality** means being in-itself with a unique interiority, privacy and inner self. **Relationality** is being towards-others with self-possession, self-communication and self-transcendence.

Mutual Goal Setting

It is a foundational thought of this text that caring for the health needs of a community requires a unified set of disciplines focused on excellent clinical behaviors with the goal of health. Health-care organizations are communities, relational social systems, whose proper end or goal is increasing the health of those who come within the organization's care as patients, clients, or employees. We have discussed human nature and being a person in the contemporary Aristotelian perspective of Clarke. It is believed that Philosophy becomes accessible to practitioners through theory that brings together relevant philosophical beliefs and knowledge of practice to facilitate clinical decisions. Here, we take a moment to consider how this philosophical perspective of human nature can guide practice. The nursing educator and theorist, Imogene King (1923 – 2007) affirmed in a private conversation February 24, 2004 that although written for nursing, the concepts and processes of interactions and transactions for setting mutual goals apply to all health-care disciplines. Put simply, King's theory asserts that mutually established goals will result in better outcomes than standardized instructions or telling patients what they ought to do for their self-care. King studied the philosophy of Thomas Aquinas as an undergraduate and his Aristotelian view of humanity is at the core of

---

[61] Clark, p.4.
[62] Clark, p.14-15.

the personal system within her conceptual framework for practice.[63]

The Health-care Setting as Permeable Systems

King's conceptual framework organizes the complex health-care setting into three interlocking permeable systems: the personal system, the interpersonal system and the social system.[64] The personal system, the core of health-care, captures the substantial physical individual, body and soul. The practitioner and patient enter into dialogue and interaction within the interpersonal system. These transcendent health-care activities, and all health care, occur within social systems. "King operationalized within a nursing context what Aristotle taught about being human. Passages expressing the importance of empowering patients to make decisions and participate in mutual goal setting reflect the uniquely human capacity of conceptual knowledge and the capacity of making choices based on that knowledge."[65] Let me re-emphasize that in personal communication, King said even though she could not develop the concepts at this time, the framework and theory were applicable to all health-care disciplines. This is reasonable given that the foundation of her work is a philosophical understanding of human nature.

In 2007 Whelton wrote, "Mobility, appetites, and many emotions are shared with other animals. However, the desire for knowledge and goodness (excellent living) are uniquely human as appetites of the intellect. These are capacities of the will. Human freedom is making choices based on knowledge of situations and principles or laws within the situations. Without knowledge there is no real freedom. The capacity for shared knowledge, requiring immaterial concepts and language, is unique to human life."[66]

"A treatment plan with mutually set goals respects the humanity and,

---

[63] King, I. "King's Structure, Process, and Outcome in the 21st Century," in *Middle Range Theory Development Using King's Conceptual System,* Christina Leibold Sieloff and Maureen Fry (editors), New York: Springer Publishing Company, 2007, pp. 3-11, esp. p.8.

[64] King provides the Personal System Concepts: Self, Growth and Development, Body Image, Space, Time, Learning, and Perception. King's Interpersonal System Concepts are Interaction, Communication, Transactions, Role, and Stress. King provides the Social System concepts of Organization, Authority, Power, Status, and Decision Making.

[65] Whelton, 2007, p.17-18.

[66] Whelton, 2007, p.18.

thus, the inherent dignity of the human person."[67]....As a student of human nature, King recognized that human action requires knowledge and freedom: "health professionals have a responsibility to share information that helps individuals make informed decisions about their health."[68] Notice that the caregiver has the responsibility to share knowledge with the client and to develop options into a treatment plan in–collaboration with the client. This mutuality of knowledge and shared vision is critical for therapeutic transactions in King's theory of goal attainment. In 1981, King wrote, "working together they [the nurse and patient] experience a new kind of relationship in the health care system, one in which the patient is recognized as having a part in making decisions that affect him now and, in the future, and is recognized as a person whose participation gives him some independence and control in the situation."[69]

Conclusion

Substantial form makes an individual the kind of being that it is. In human development, this energizing principle gives rise to the primary properties essential to being human. Substances have a principle of individuation and change (matter) and a principle of universality and stability (form). It is form that is known when humans know the world. Human knowing moves beyond the problem-solving capacities of animals because of the ability to think about and to reason from immaterial concepts organized into sentences and propositions used as premises and conclusions of arguments.

When something is known it can be desired or avoided. Since desire energizes and moves to action, limiting knowledge limits choices. Human freedom requires knowledge of options and the physical and emotional freedom to act on the known options. As animals we share with all animals the characteristic of sensitive life. But as human, we must add the rational capacities of intellect and will. The intellectual ability to abstract immaterial concepts from perceptions gained through experience provides the most characteristic, essential capacity of human life. This highest human capacity is respected when one provides knowledge needed for personal choice. Knowledge of how humans can live a harmonious productive life is the professional caregiver's interface with virtue, and the

---

[67] Whelton, B. J. B., (1999). The philosophical core of Imogene King's behavioral system. *Nursing Science Quarterly*, 12 (2), 158-163.

[68] King, I. M. (1981). *A theory for nursing: Systems, concepts, processes.* New York: Wiley. p. 144.

[69] King, 1981, p.86.

moral foundations for ethical decision making.

Norris Clarke's classic and contemporary descriptions teach that humans are matter-form unities, substantial beings, whose relationality and self-transcendence takes one into communion with others. As relational social beings we participate in the world connecting ourselves to others in families, friendships, and communities. We gain our self-awareness from the way we are treated by significant persons in our interpersonal environment. Our receptivity to others leads to loving self-transcendence, which is an overflowing of self towards others

We considered accounts of Quinlan and Schiavo as persons in community. We shared the growth of the health-care community as it learned to care for unconscious patients and their families. We were confronted with the distinction of removing equipment (extra-ordinary care) so that a person may die and not feeding (ordinary care) so that one will die.

We also saw that a comatose individual retains the right to refuse medical interventions through their previously created documentation or the expression of wishes made by the surrogate decision maker. Finally, we were introduced to King's theoretical work that extends philosophical insights of the human person into clinical practice.

Conversation Starters:

1. Use the distinctions of matter and form, essential and accidental properties (attributes) to describe a friend in class. You can do this for each other.

2. In your understanding of human life, what is the source of human dignity? What calls us to treat each other with respect?

3. Virtue is said to be a human excellence, a superior condition of the soul. What if there is no soul? Then, what is human excellence? How does one evaluate human excellence?

4. Define concepts and provide examples of concepts that remain the same and concepts that are ever changing.

5. We say human persons are to be treated with respect. Yet this does not always happen.

   a. Describe a time when you clearly felt you were being treated as a person.

   b. Describe a time when you clearly felt you were being treated as a thing. What could have been done to transform this situation into one with you feeling like a person.

Reflection Submissions:

1. Provide your answer and use arguments to support your position, why do humans exist? What is the end or purpose of human life?

2. It has been asserted that concepts are immaterial, if so the mind which reasons with these immaterial concepts is immaterial. If you were to argue that humans have an immaterial capacity, the mind, what is the source of this immateriality? If you were to argue that humans do not have an immaterial capacity, what is the mind?

3. Consider the mystery of human life: Who am I? Who are you? Who are we? Here are some descriptors to include: a soul, a body, a thing, an embodied spirit, a person, a potential, a complex of relationships. There are others you may think of. It is important that you support the selection of your descriptors from thought and experience. A paragraph or two is expected. Everyone writes their own paper. You may discuss content with a classmate. Please provide their name as a reference in your paper.

Outline for Chapter 4: Humans as Persons in Community
A. Properties of Human Nature
   1. Humans as the knowing subject (knower)
      a. The senses
      b. Human intellectual capacities
      c. The will as appetite
   2. An Excellent Human Life
      a. Respect for others
   3. Characteristic Capacities of Beings
   4. Humans are the Rational Animals
      a. Aquinas on immateriality
      b. Health and virtue
      c. Social beings
      d. Self-consciousness
   5. Sleeping Beauty
B. Lessons from Quinlan and Schiavo
   1. Cure may be futile, but care never futile.
   2. Terri Schiavo
   3. Right to refuse medical interventions
C. Knowing and Choice are the Basis of Self-determination
   1. All life is worth living; some interventions are not worth having
   2. Humans as substantial, relational, and transcendent
D. Mutual Goal Setting
   1. The health-care setting as permeable systems
E. Conclusion

Terminology for Chapter 4
Essential
Accidental
Self-transcendence
Outer senses
Inner senses
Cognitive
Estimative
Modally distinct
Intellect
Will
Health
Virtue
Knowing

Percept
Autonomy
Informed consent
Paternalism
Substantiality
Relationality

SECTION THREE:

PERSONS

CHAPTER 5

THE PRACTITIONER IS FIRST A HUMAN
AND THEN A PROFESSIONAL

Objectives

Upon completion of this chapter you will be able to:

1. Make use of values in discussions and writings about life and practice.
2. Explain how ethical practice requires a virtuous practitioner.
3. Demonstrate how human excellence sets limits on behavior.
4. Compare and contrast the healing act and the moral act.

Two Ancient Parables

The Ring of Gyges

Considering the self as an individual and as a professional brings to mind two ancient parables. One is in Plato's Republic (Book II, 359b-360c), The Ring of Gyges;[70] the other in the New Testament biblical scriptures, Luke 15: 11-32,[71] the Prodigal Son. Since Plato's account is older, we consider it first. The *Republic* tells the story of a discussion between Plato's mentor, Socrates, and some young men, including the Sophist, Thrasymachus, and Plato's brother Glaucon. Sophists are interesting figures in the history of ideas. They are the first known teachers selling a particular curriculum and receiving payment. They went city to city in ancient Greece teaching young men how to argue well. They were generally not concerned with the truth or falsity of a position. They wanted to win the argument. This was important because an accused citizen, that

---

[70] Plato's Republic. Translated by G.M.A. Grube. Indianapolis: Hackett Publishing Company, 1974.
[71] The New American Bible for Catholics, Australia, 1986.

is a land-owning male, had to defend himself in court. There were no lawyers.

Justice as a Virtue

The discussion of the *Republic* is in search of the accurate definition of justice. I like to think the virtue justice is meant, but there are legal and political meanings as well. In the first book of the *Republic*, Thrasymachus proposes that justice is the advantage of the stronger. In other words, justice was of no value unless a person used it to his own advantage. Justice had been tentatively defined by Plato early in the discussion as "to give to each their due." In the ancient culture this meant doing well towards your friends and evil towards your enemies. Even today we are left saying, "What is due to whom?"

Plato's brother Glaucon takes up Thrasymachus's sophistic position in Book II. He argued better than being just was to appear just while actually being unjust. He supports this position with a parable. Gyges was in the service of the King. He was hired to care for the sheep. Shall we call him a 'professional' sheep herder? One afternoon, Gyges is tending sheep in an ancient fertile valley. In an earthquake the land opens and reveals a corpse within an ornate hollow bronze horse. Fascinated by the vision, and uncertain of its reality, Gyges takes the ring from the dead soldier's finger. Sometime later, he discovers that turning the ring one way made him invisible. Those in attendance continue speaking, but now as if he were not present. He turns the ring the other way, and those present include him in their conversation. The shepherd earned a position as messenger for the king. With his newly found power of invisibility, he stole whatever he wanted, committed adultery with the queen, killed the king and took over the kingdom. The argument is that, given the opportunity, this is what any person would do. It would be foolish to do otherwise. Being a just person has no meaning because sometimes the good person suffers, and those who do evil prosper. One's reputation is what is important and a reputation for being just was only worthwhile when used to your own advantage.

Pulling this Parable Forward to our Time

When people act anonymously in a group or more famously "behind the corporate veil," utilizing legal protections from incorporation of a company, they may act in their own self-interest without regard for others. Many health-care practitioners rightfully incorporate their practice to protect their assets. The corporation is a legal person with legal rights and responsibilities in acquiring debt, entering into contracts, paying out profits, paying taxes, suing and being sued, and so on. We are not asserting a negative attitude toward incorporation. It is the right thing to do. Difficulties emerge when those involved see incorporation as an opportunity to act anonymously and, thus, without accountability.

The online legal dictionary says, "The rights and responsibilities of a corporation are independent and distinct from the people who own or invest in them. A corporation simply provides a way for individuals to run a business and to share in profits and losses."[72] Because of misuse of this separation between an incorporated business and the actual persons making decisions and benefiting from their protections, the corporate veil is said to have been pierced to hold officers and stockholders accountable.[73] The decisions of a corporation are nothing more than the decisions of its board of directors. Corporations do not make decisions, people do. Therefore the law was rewritten to hold people, not corporations, responsible.

Applying Lessons from The Ring of Gyges

Health professional applications of lessons from the parable of the Ring of Gyges include the reason specific team members are assigned to specific responsibilities. Usually a task or opportunity assigned to all never gets done. Another application is seen in the care of persons clearly unable to report abuse or neglect. The anonymity of the care giver in the care of the elderly nursing home resident or vulnerable disabled child enhances the potential for abuse or neglect. The mentally ill are likewise vulnerable because it is hard to sort the real from the imagined in their accounts. These persons can be abused with no one knowing it happened, or if it is discovered there is usually no way to trace who did it.

Virtue of Justice is Doing What Ought to be Done When No One Knows It

Professionals have to maintain proper care because they are committed to these good actions and not because their behaviors are known or unknown. Another way of saying this is to note that professional practice

---

[72] http://legal-dictionary.thefreedictionary.com/Corporate+veil (accessed March 16, 2013)
[73] http://nationalparalegal.edu/public_documents/courseware_asp_files/business Law/Directors%26Officers/PiercingCorporateVeil.asp (accessed July 30 2015)

in health care requires human excellence. Again, virtue is doing what ought to be done when no one knows it.

As professional practitioners, the parable ought not to apply, but it does not take too much imagination to see theft from insurance companies as the reverse application of the lesson. Practitioners do not perceive themselves as taking from individuals when they falsify records to expand charges to insurance companies. They would never steal from another person, but stealing from an insurance company is different. No particular known persons are involved. It needs to be emphasized that these insurance funds are taken from people. An insurance company is a community of people.

The Prodigal Son

It may seem peculiar that a text on health-care ethics would relate the parable of the prodigal son, but there is a very interesting line that contrasts with the shepherd in the Ring of Gyges. This parable is the account of a young man who wants to leave his father's house and make his own way in the world. He asks his father for the money equivalent to his anticipated inheritance. The father complies, gives him his fortune, and the son sets out for a distant country. In his new-found wealth and freedom, he parties. The New American Bible says, "he squandered his inheritance on a life of dissipation (Luke 15: 13)." The King James Version says, "The younger son gathered all together, and took his journey into a far country, and there wasted his substance with riotous living." Famously, while caring for pigs, a despised animal in Jewish culture, he comes to his senses and goes home where his father receives him with great joy. The line we want to consider is verse 16: "And he longed to eat his fill of the pods on which the swine fed, but nobody gave him any."

Pulling this Parable Forward to Our Time

This young man was motivated to return home to work for his father by his extreme hunger. He was starving, but he would not eat what was not given to him. How many of us would feel it would have been acceptable to take some of the animal's food to not starve? In my understanding, the pods were corn husks; surely he could have found some clean corn to eat. We can take from this parable that although he was foolish and self-centered, he was honest. It is true, he would ask his father for his inheritance long before it was due to him, but he would not take corn from his employer. We note that he did not just take what was essentially his from his father without asking. It could be said that somewhere deep within this young man there was an awareness of who he was and a sense of honesty; a truthfulness that guided his actions.

Meaning from the Parables

Both of these parables display for us a deeper meaning, perhaps different from the original. The account of Gyges provides a glimpse into how a working person can get caught up in inappropriate or unjust behavior. I know of people who have taken what they thought were fantastic well-paying positions only to find the primary practitioner, dentist or physician, was involved in illegal activity. To preserve their values they chose to find another job. The parable of the prodigal son might mean that a person's deeper character (virtue) can call him back from horrible mistakes. Each one of us has or will make mistakes. One of the purposes of this book is to encourage you to know your values and consider your responsibilities in order to spare you from mistakes others have made.

As health-care practitioners we are each one vulnerable. We have to know our strengths and weaknesses. Of course, we want to build on our strengths and avoid our weaknesses. For example, if you have a tendency toward addiction, do not take a position where narcotics are easily available. Being honest with yourself and preventing temptations is much better than trying to repair your career, even though it can be done. The prodigal son did go home, but did he have to come to the point of starvation? He could have been adventurous and traveled but also acted with a bit more wisdom; taking the moderate road.

Caring for the Self

In a way, this chapter is about the practitioner's responsibility to himself or herself. One must engage in self-care to maintain the substantial person; the matter-form unity we spoke of in previous chapters. Within your work you need to maintain body, soul, and essential relationships with family and community.

Consider the impact of long hours and shift work on body rhythms, eating, and sleeping. Within the hospital and nursing home, care is required around the clock, but health-care professionals have a responsibility to themselves, colleagues, and their patients to maintain their strength and capacity to make good decisions and to act on them. One needs to know when they are drowsy and not be working alone at that time. Working nights, the LPN and Nurses Aid might each take a 30-minute nap in the staff room rather than a lunch break. Almost everyone has a drowsy time. It is better to know that this is the case and accommodate. However, the nurse in charge cannot take a nap.

You need a plan for getting the sleep, fluids, and food you need as a physical being. There was an excellent nurse who also had three teen-aged children. Asked how she managed the energy demands of her life, she said one 24-hour period every month she stayed in bed. Her family cared for themselves and for her. She said the teens took pride in planning this day. What are your creative solutions? There is also a professional responsibility to be prepared to serve patients.

One afternoon, I was with my sister as she was being admitted to a hospital. This was a pretty routine admission. The nurse who came to do the intake was exhausted. She fell asleep a couple of times doing the required paperwork. She said she had worked a double shift when asked if she were okay. I worried if she had gotten the information accurate. There seemed little I could do as family member observing the situation. I asked if someone else could finish the questions. She said no that she had to finish the admission before she could go home. She excused herself and came back a bit more alert and finished her assignment. What if you are in this condition when an emergency occurs, be that four in the morning or four in the afternoon? Are you depending on an adrenaline rush? All health practitioners face difficult situations when they or a colleague is unsafe to practice because of lack of sleep, drugs, or illness. As a professional you are called to practice a healthy life style and to be alert to your needs, so you do not become vulnerable to neglect of your duties. What if your coworker, doing lab work or CAT scans or sonograms, exhibits inappropriate behavior? Is it different if they are ill or overtired, or if they are intoxicated or high on drugs?

We are physical beings, and this is never more apparent than when we are incapacitated. Our emotional and intellectual responses are impaired when our physiology is disrupted. Professional education, more than other academic curricula, is interested in development of the professional person as well as the knowledge within the discipline. When you come to a patient as a respiratory therapist or dental hygienist, you enable that person to share their need for the kind of care appropriate to your discipline. When approaching the patient (one who is vulnerable), the caregiver brings their preparation and their desire to assist, but they also bring the stresses and incapacities (issues they did not resolve).

The Healing Act[74]

Health settings are like communities. One could say within an ideal health-care setting there are multiple practitioners seeking to assist patients with the knowledge and skills they bring to the situation. Within this community setting, the healing actions are exchanges between individuals in which one person is enriched in their quest for health by the presence and abilities of another. In the perspective of this text, dying is a natural end of living. There is still wholeness or health in ones dying.

This healing exchange, at the heart of health care, is a moral act calling a practitioner to be a person of virtue. That is, one who has cared for himself, has habits of acting well, and is prepared and willing to serve the patients. Both moral actions and healing actions are grounded in what it is to be human. They are within a larger class of behavior called human actions like eating well, sleeping enough, studying, playing, and walking. Even though involving physical needs, these activities are chosen and freely carried out as one's own. If we were to use a set of circles, we would say the outer ring was composed of these human actions. Inside human actions are excellent actions additionally specified as moral by their excellence and emphasis on the human good. The healing act is among the multiple moral actions that can be performed. The human act, the moral act, and the healing act share a common structure and fit together. The moral act is an excellent human act with the healing act being a subset of the moral act. These purposeful professional healing behaviors require knowledge, experience, capacity, and an intention toward the good of health.

Culture of Integrity

Continuing with our idealized vision, we can say human excellence is found in discerning the best action to be done in a situation, choosing to do the action, and then doing the good action. This moral excellence is found in an action characterized as a principle-based action performed as good for another and as the agent's own good. Notice the emphasis on "the agent's own good." This is saying, what I do that is good for you is, in

---

[74] These ideas are summarized from, Whelton, B.J. "The Nursing Act is an Excellent Human Act: A Philosophical Analysis Derived from Classical Philosophy and the Conceptual Framework and Theory of Imogene King," Chapter Two, *Middle Range Theory Development Using King's Conceptual System,* Christina Leibold Sieloff and Maureen Fry (editors), New York: Springer Publishing Company, 2007, pp. 12-28.

fact, good for me. This good is my human fulfillment. In this there is an identifiable interpersonal transaction or exchange that brings healing to the recipient and fulfillment to the healer. We are saying this giving act of the practitioner is an excellence of soul and, thus, moral action. There is a sense in which the whole healing community of caregivers requires and develops a culture of integrity. Clearly, this is the expression of an unattainable ideal, but perhaps a goal that guides our efforts just as the perfect person does not exist except as an ideal.

In sum, as emerging from the humanity of the practitioner, the healing act is a human act. As a human excellence, the healing act is a moral act requiring that one be disposed to see the good to be done and have the discipline to do it. As a part of the therapeutic community, the healing act is an interpersonal transaction that focuses directly on the patient's well-being (individual, family or community) but gives back personal fulfillment and communion within the community.

The Healing Act is a Moral Act

Robert Sokolowski, in his analysis, *The Moral Act: A Phenomenological Study*[75] stresses the interpersonal character of moral action in holding that a moral act is a transaction in which another's good becomes my good in these circumstances. It is essential, however, that the practitioner be able to see both the truth of the patient's need and their responsibility to act to alleviate or fill this need. The practitioner must also have the perseverance and courage to do what is now known to be required by the patient's situation. This acting to meet the patient's need as good for the patient is moral (as the moral action). Additionally, fulfilling the good of the other is experienced as the practitioner's own good. One of Sokolowski's important insights is the reflexivity of the moral act. Morality is not just giving of one's self. When I act for your good, it is also good for me.

In a course paper, written about healing actions, I wrote that the nursing act is the nurse acting for the good of the patient as his or her good for the patient. Sokolowski crossed through "for the patient." What do you think? Was he right? Could it be, if the caregiver acts only for the good of the patient the caregiver will feel drained by their practice? Are they apt to experience "burn out"?

Reflecting on these questions, I found that my good for the other must also be good for me as the fulfillment of who I am. If healing is a moral

---

[75] Bloomington: Indiana University Press, 1985, esp. Ch. 3 "Moral Action".

act, as here proposed, it is an excellence, the fulfillment of one's self as human as well as the fulfillment of one's self as health-care practitioner. When my actions are done for the good of another's health, these actions fulfill who I am as physician, nurse, therapist or technician. I am energized rather than fatigued. At the end of the day, the healers may be physically exhausted, but when their actions have expressed who they are, there will also be an energized satisfaction, even joy, at having served well.

Sokolowski's Healing Exchange

This synthesis of being and doing in the healing exchange is seen in Sokolowski's description of medicine and the physician. He writes,

> Because the art of medicine aims at something that is a good for the patient, the doctor, in the exercise of his art, seeks the medical good of the patient as his own good....The nature of his art, with the perspectives it provides on the medical good, gives the physician this harmony, and it makes him, in the good exercise of his art, not only a good doctor but also essentially a good moral agent, one who seeks the good of another formally as his own. The doctor's profession essentially makes him a good man, provided he is true to his art and follows its insistence.[76]

Expanding Sokolowski's Insight of the Healing Exchange

It is the position of this text that all of the healing arts are moral practices in their application of health knowledge specific to the practitioner who is encountering a vulnerable person enabling him or her to receive healing within the practitioner's discipline and the patient's need. Additionally, the practitioner grows in morality when he or she practices the healing art of their discipline.

Heath care is very complex with multiple practitioners and specialists, technologies, and third party payers. Much of the health-care enterprise does not fall within the above conception of the healing act. Many interventions are removing impediments or making a way for nature to restore itself within the patient. A personal healing interaction may not be required, or patients get better in spite of its absence. There are also a number of activities of health-care providers that are not directly related to healing. In addition to human resources, there is much technology to manage, and a business to run. These are intended for the end of health; but in themselves, they do not heal. They set up environments in which

---

[76] "The Art and Science of Medicine," in *Catholic Perspectives on Medical Morals: Foundational Issues,* E.D. Pellegrino, J.P. Langan, and J.C. Harvey, eds. Dordrecht: Kluwer Academic Publishers, 1989, 263-275. (p. 269)

practitioners can care for patients. With all of its complexity, at center core health care is human interactions that heal. The healing agent is the person who gives of him or herself to the patient as the agent's own good.

Informal Healer

Healing that is being placed at the core of the therapeutic relationship (between practitioner and patient) is not exclusive to the healing professions. Some say the bartender is the best therapist. He or she is an **informal healer,** if what is needed is a listening ear and someone who acknowledges the personal pain of the patron. The difficulty with this scenario is the mix with alcohol that can generate more pain rather than healing.

Another setting is the nurturance of maternal caring. A nurturing mother detects her child's need as an opportunity to give of herself for the child's good. This is the fulfillment of herself as person and as mother.

All persons working within a health-care setting can have a healing presence, even the housekeeper or maintenance staff. Sometimes the chaplain is the most important healer by resolving spiritual conflicts and strengthening the individual so that their energy can be focused on becoming healthy again or peacefully living until death occurs.

These healing actions are not acts of friendship. They are not among equals, and there is not a mutual sharing of stories; one person needs to have the capacity to meet the need of the other. Need becomes vulnerability in the recipient, and the capacity to meet this need awakens responsibility in the healer and is also a source of power. This power differential is the inequality in the relationship and demands virtue within the professional to not take advantage of the vulnerable. Not all aspects of the caregiver-patient relationship and not all behaviors of health-care providers are healing actions. Healing actions are unique interpersonal transactions which move the patient towards health and the caregiver is energized and affirmed in his or her vocation as healer.

Seedhouse's Exposition of Caring Actions

Professor David Seedhouse, of Auckland, New Zealand,[77] has studied questions of caring in health care for many years. From his research he identifies four meanings of caring in health care. While Seedhouse's work

---

[77] *Practical Nursing Philosophy:The Universal Ethical Code.* Chichester, West Sussex: John Wiley & Sons, LTD, 2000. {p. 33-39).

was done within nursing, I suspect it is transferable to all caring disciplines. It explains that the technicians or technologists, who do their assignments with accuracy and precision, with or without personal emotion, are caring for the patient even when the patient does not feel cared about.

Seedhouse first provides from the work of Watson[78] and of Noddings[79] that caring is a tenderness requiring personal involvement and deep empathetic relationships, typical of feminine practitioners. He then challenges that emotional involvement is not necessary for care and is insufficient to answer difficult questions. Intellectual analysis is still required.

The second type of caring is the practical performance of activities required of a sick person and doing them properly. This care can be provided to the ill without emotional involvement. One does not need to even like the person cared for. There may be a sense of duty but not tenderness.

The third type of caring is associated with good judgment. The practitioner shows this good judgment in selecting and providing activities identified as most likely to provide good outcomes. These activities would be within the practitioner's discipline and prescribed by the ordering physician. This reasoning and intervention does not require direct personal involvement, just the desire to intervene effectively.

The final, and fourth, type of caring is service done for the sake of the one who receives interventions but has no relationship to tenderness or involvement. The one caring portrays a personal interest where it does not exist because the recipient needs to think they are personally cared about. This is presented as a professional skill, a craft.[80] The practitioner pretends to be concerned when they are not; they are actually distracted by personal problems or school work. He or she may act pleasant when really, they are depressed or angry. One could think there is a loss of integrity pretending you are happy when you are not. But, think about it, you have a job to do and you were hired for that job. Professional practitioners are not allowed to 'call in' and not work just because they are irritated and cannot honestly portray a peaceful interior. One's mood may even lighten as clients are served.

---

[78] Watson, J., "Human caring and suffering: a subjective model for health sciences," in *They Shall Not Hurt: Human Suffering and Human Caring,* ed. R. Taylor and J. Watson, Colorado Associated University Press 1989.

[79] Noddings, N. *Caring: A Feminist Approach to Ethics and Moral Education,* Berkely: University of California Press, 1984.

[80] Seedhouse, p.38.

Being Professional

Professionals are people set aside by society to fulfill necessary roles. The professional has a unique body of knowledge; an acknowledged status in the community, rights, and responsibilities; and the authority to fulfill one's professional role. As a professional there is moral guidance from codes of practice, and state licensure solidifies the warrant to practice and establishes legal parameters.

The professional is expected to uphold high personal standards and has certain immunities and protections in performing prescribed duties. For example, physicians and nurses are protected from accusations of impropriety in the legitimate performance of examinations, intimate hygienic measures, and treatments. Medical assistants are trusted to prepare patients for physical examinations. The ultrasound and radiology technicians need to also maintain professional behavior and are similarly protected in their physical measures for development of scans. Health care is an intimate practice requiring virtue on the part of practitioners, especially with frightened seductive patients.

Multifaceted Healing Practice

Healing practice is multifaceted involving principles and practices of health-care sciences and researchers who work in the sciences, as well as practitioners who use knowledge from research to achieve effective healing situations. In a rather bold way we have asserted that humanity, the universal understanding of human life found in both the recipient of care and the caregiver, is the foundation of moral health care practices. The humanity of the practitioner and of the patient is the core of health-care sciences as well as the practice arts. As with clinical practice, this foundation of health care in the humanity of patient and practitioner is true for most health-care disciplines and therapies.

Actions are on the level of the particular. One gives medication to a particular patient. One enters into a healing transaction with an individual in their circumstances with their family and community. How can there be a healing science for respiratory therapy, nuclear medicine, or health information management? Where is the scientific knowledge; the universal content? Whether you accept scientific knowledge as stable universal content or generalizations from data leading to likely accounts or confirmed beliefs, scientific knowledge is generally considered to be the results of research. Health-care science provides a stable base of organized knowledge generated by documented controlled inquiry. Science is not individual particular interventions. These are the art of practice. In addition to these facets of science and art, professional health disciplines have technologies and areas of active discipline-specific research.

The Distinction between Speculative and Practical Scientists

The speculative scientist analyzes effects and does research to uncover the principles and causes of the effects. The goal of truly speculative inquiry is just to have knowledge. Research is conducted in order to uncover and then support that the object of inquiry actually exists or that identified principles are in fact the causes of specified effects. In drawing conclusions and publishing studies, the speculative scientist may compose logical proofs confirming results, but the method of speculative science is primarily analysis.[81]

Similarly, the practical scientist will analyze and study materials, behaviors, or desired effects in order to discover their principles and causes. Nevertheless, the practical scientist is not primarily concerned with truth about nature. The study does not conclude with the composition of a proof and publication of a report, although these are important. The goal of practical inquiry is the discovery of principles and actions appropriate for the achievement of desired ends. These principles of action are practical truths. In a practice discipline, the researcher, just as the clinician, is seeking to know what is needed and correct in order to generate a cure or improved health. Health-care researchers inquire into behaviors that represent both responses to interventions and interventions themselves. Researchers identify and support principles and causes that explain patient responses or support certain behaviors as the correct thing to do for prevention of illness, curing disease, or the promotion or production of the fullness of human life captured in the word 'health.'

Practical science does not generate a situation or a product. Science provides knowledge of principles and causes for the practitioner who must carefully assess and evaluate a particular situation. Practical sciences are completed by practitioners, not as science but as art, be that political arts, engineering arts, healing arts or therapeutic arts. This art of practice does not just refer to skills. The art of clinical practice is the skillful, experienced application of disciplinary knowledge within particular situations. Practitioners require good judgment (wisdom) in the use of

---

[81] Wallace, W.A. *From a Realist Point of View: Essays on the Philosophy of Science*, 2nd ed. Lanham: University Press of America,1983. Ch 13 "Being Scientific in a Practice Discipline."

principles acquired from learning the accepted body of knowledge. These principles are used in the composition of interventions towards the end of health. Medical, nursing, respiratory therapy or principles of testing may be acquired from speculative, productive, and practical disciplines or from primary research within the discipline itself. Research inquiring into principles from other disciplines, like cellular biology, imports them into the organized body of therapeutic knowledge, but only if their explanatory and prescriptive value is confirmed in the discipline using the content.

A professional practitioner has available the body of knowledge learned as disciplinary science. In a particular patient interaction, principles are selected, applied, even modified to compose a response to intervene in the patient situation. This composition of a healing situation is the practitioner's art.[82] The therapeutic art of practice is the professional seeing and meeting the needs of the individual as the practitioner's good for this patient in this situation. This interaction is the setting within which healing occurs. Thus, the healing act is a moral transaction grounded in the humanity of both practitioner and patient, and the professional practitioner's good practice.

Conclusion

The above descriptions confront the humanity of the practitioner and the patient's need for self-care as well as what the professional contributes. This chapter asserted that the healing act is a moral act. If it also carries the attributes and responsibilities of a moral act, there are significant implications for understanding effective health-care interventions as requiring the practitioner to be virtuously disposed towards the patient's good in order to grasp both the principles and particulars in a situation requiring intervention. Without a virtuous disposition, an individual would not see the good of the other as his or her own good, bringing self-fulfillment as an individual and as a practitioner. This interpersonal core makes the practice of the health-care professional a moral practice.

---

[82] Pellegrino writes, "Medicine comes into existence *qua* medicine only when scientific knowledge is focused on a decision that is good for a particular patient." "Science and Theology: From a Medical Perspective," *Linacre Quarterly,* November 1990, 19-34. (p. 23). See also, "Ethics and the Moral Center of the Medical Enterprise" *Bulletin of the New York Academy of Medicine,* July-August 1978 (54:7) 625-639.

Conversation Starters:
1. Is not telling the truth you know different from lying to cover over the truth you know. Describe a time, if any, when it's right to lie. Identify a time, if any, when it's right to not tell the truth. Is there a value higher than truth-telling?
2. Does it make a difference if your co-worker is ill or overtired, or if they are intoxicated or high on drugs? Under which of these circumstances would you notify the supervisor? Why?
3. Student athletes are not allowed to drink 48 hours before a game. Why are adults allowed to have one or two mixed drinks and then drive? Consider the difference. What is needed for working adults to be safe on the job?

Reflection Submissions:
1. Define and provide an example of each of the classic cardinal virtues (wisdom, courage, moderation and justice) as private individual and as health care professional. Be sure to begin with defining virtue and the virtues, then provide the examples. Finally, write a reflection on similarities and differences.
2. Consideration of student's disciplinary code of ethics: Obtain a copy of the Code of Ethics for a health-care discipline of your choice. These are available on-line by looking for the code of ethics for your discipline or one closely related. Write short answers and support for your answers to the following questions (using in your paper specific items from your code as evidence):
   a.) Does it include your relationship with other members of the profession?
   b.) Does it provide for the continuance of the discipline?
   c.) Does it address what treatment is within the purview of the discipline?
   d.) What are the dominant themes and positions promoted in the code?
   e.) Does it address human rights? In what way?
   f.) Does it provide content needed to resolve an ethical situation into an optimum action?

Support your answer.

Outline for Chapter 5: The Practitioner is First a Human Then a Professional
A. Two Ancient Parables
  1. The Ring of Gyges
      a. Justice as a virtue
      b. Pulling this parable forward to our time
      c. Applying lessons from The Ring of Gyges
      d. Virtue of Justice is doing what ought to be done when no one knows it.
  2. The Prodigal Son
      a. Pulling this parable forward to our time
  3. Meaning from the parables
B. Caring for the Self
C. The Healing Act
  1. Culture of integrity
D. The Healing Act as a Moral Act
  1. Sokolowski's Healing Exchange
      a. Expanding Sokolowski's insight of the healing exchange
  2. Informal healer
E. Seedhouse's Exposition of Caring Actions
F. Being Professional
  1. Multifaceted healing practice
  2. The distinction between speculative and practical scientists
G. Conclusion

Terminology for Chapter 5
Integrity
Human act
Moral act
Healing act
Justice
justice
Professional
Caring
Health-care science
Health-care arts

CHAPTER 6

THE PATIENT IS ALSO A PERSON

Objectives

This chapter provides an opportunity for the student to:

1. Describe sources and impact of patient vulnerability.
2. Relate patient vulnerability to the moral responsibilities of the practitioner.
3. Describe international codes to protect vulnerable subjects.
4. Acknowledge human requirements for knowledge and freedom.
5. Describe Natural Law ethics and the guidance provided for moral decisions.

The Patient is First a Human Being

To say "the patient is also a person," is to mean the individual is more than a patient or client for the practice of my specialty or yours. This individual, presenting for care, is at the same time, his or her own person. This individual, couple, or family has a history of events and relationships that brought them to this point in their life. Aristotle and Aquinas in their discussion of virtue, Hegel and Sartre in their discussion of human development taught whatever and whomever one is today is the result of a history of daily decisions, small and large. Additionally, this brief time with you, as a professional, includes the patient's future and is the beginning of who they will be whether individual, family, or community. It is your moment to increase or decrease their inner strength, abilities, and hope. Some might say, "Don't put that on me." Or you reply, "I'm just doing a scan or X-ray, or giving a treatment." It is simple, but the human interchange is inevitable. Your presentation, affect, and attitude will make a difference; there is no indifference within this moral moment. Even though you may choose to treat the other with indifference, they will be impacted by your presence.

In the philosophical perspective of the human person discussed in Chapters Three and Four, the patient is a substantial being, a physical matter form unity in their own transcendent context that includes their being within family, community, health-care environment, and their own way of being in the world. Even if you are with the patient for only a few minutes, providing excellent health care requires that you see and support the integrity of the individual and address the whole person. I have never met "the upper GI in room three" or "Dr. Stern's patient in room 246." You will probably use these expressions for ease of speaking in the clinical area, but at least for this time, I want you to think of how it objectifies and distances you from your patient. Although current HIPPA laws require patients not be publicly addressed by name, when speaking directly with the patients, using their names enhances the relationship.

Vulnerability

The Council for International Organizations of Medical Sciences (CIOMS) in the *International Ethical Guidelines for Biomedical Research involving human subjects (2002)* describes vulnerability as follows: "Vulnerable persons are those who are relatively (or absolutely) incapable of protecting their own interests. More formally, they may have insufficient power, intelligence, education, resources, strength, or other needed attributes to protect their own interests."[83] This reads like a list of incapacities for which health-care professionals intervene:

Powerlessness calling for advocacy;
Lack of knowledge calling for health education;
Lack of resources calling for social interventions;
Intellectual and physical incapacity calling for physical care and advocacy.

In her 2003 discussion of international research in the journal *Bioethics,* Ruth Macklin interprets the above quotation to say, "The chief characteristic of vulnerability that this guideline identifies is a limited capacity or freedom to consent or to decline to participate in research."[84] (And, let us add, health-care decisions.)

---

[83] Geneva, Switzerland. Guideline 13:64.
[84] "Bioethics, Vulnerability, and Protection," *Bioethics* ISSN 0269-9702 (print); 1 467-8519 (on-line) Volume 17 Numbers5-6 2003.
http://www.unige.ch/medecine/ib/ethiqueBiomedicale/enseignement/programmeY 2006/me-12-Macklin-vulnerability-and-protection.pdf (accessed June 10, 2013)

Vulnerability Follows Injury and Illness

Not knowing what is wrong and how to care for one's self with an injury or illness leads the individual to expose himself, to reveal his need. It transforms the person into a potential patient (in some locations the person is a client or customer). Following the moral reasoning of Pellegrino, vulnerability in the patient generates responsibility in the one capable of intervening. But, one has to ask, does vulnerability really generate responsibility? Do you have a moral responsibility to do something just because you can? You may have asked advice of a friend who is a counselor because your granddaughter was asking for money to buy food. The counselor does not ask if she was addicted, or if she has housing, he or she just says, "If you can help, you should." Should you? Why do you hold this?

If you are an independent practitioner, do you have the right to say no; to not accept responsibility for a person's care? Conscientious objection aside, what if you just do not want to associate with this person? Generally speaking, it is considered acceptable for a physician or dentist to decide if they will treat a new patient. Once accepted, though, they are not allowed to not treat specific conditions. What about you, in your discipline, are you allowed to decline to treat someone?

Vulnerability Due to Limited Freedom

Limited freedom seems to be associated with vulnerability in all its forms. While illness and injury makes one vulnerable, limited freedom makes one more likely to suffer further injury and illness through neglect or exploitation. This discussion of vulnerability is included in this chapter because research models and evidence-based practice tend to objectify the individual. With all good intentions, obtaining results may become more important than the needs of the individual.

Consider the most vulnerable situation of an individual going into cardiac arrest right in front of you. If nothing is done, they will die. Their race, gender, education and social status are meaningless unless physiologic functioning can be restored. At this interface between life and death interventions are biochemical and physical. All persons in this situation need the same interventions to restore airway, respiration, and circulation. Achieving cardiopulmonary stability, attention can then turn to emotional and behavioral factors in the control of pain, nausea and anxiety. These interventions need to be individualized with consideration of the patient. Before discharge educational and social needs take on new significance. It is essential to include family or community organizations for effective interventions. These levels of intervention parallel the earlier discussions of the vegetative, sensitive and intellectual capacities.

Caregiver Vulnerability

In all fifty states Good Samaritan Laws protect professional and lay providers of cardio-pulmonary resuscitation (CPR). But can you be prosecuted for not doing CPR? Can you be morally excused for not intervening? For saying, "I am not responsible; it is not my duty to intervene at this time." An online document made available by the American Heart Association (2006) reports, *"If it's part of your job, you have a duty to give CPR to a victim of cardiac arrest. If it's not part of your job, you have no legal duty to give CPR. But some people think you have an ethical duty to give CPR."*[85] What do you think? Does the inherent, natural dignity of human life compel us to respond and to do so competently?

Financial and Educational Vulnerabilities

Another kind of vulnerability is seen in educational and research centers where those with limited money will often volunteer for research projects they poorly understand. It's easy to convince yourself that because few or no negative effects are discussed, there are none. Actually, this is not true. Logicians call this thinking the fallacy of ignorance when one says, "I do not know of any negative effects, so there must not be any."

Lessons of Vulnerability

The following situations are used to highlight vulnerabilities and interventions. Names and locations are fictitious except the account of John and Lynne.

Bonnie and George

Vulnerability and the inability of the staff to see it are described in the story Bonnie and George. George cares for his disabled, widowed mother,

---

[85] http://www.life1st.com/files/CPR-Legal_and_Ethical.pdf. CPR Legal and Ethical Issues. 2006.(accessed June 14, 2013)

Bonnie. Bonnie is in a wheel chair because her pelvis dissolved from loss of calcium with high doses of cortisone needed to ease symptoms of Lupus. She has been in remission but wheel chair dependent for years. Her son George is her constant companion and caregiver.

During an episode of flu, George brought his mother to the ER for uncontrolled nausea, vomiting, and diarrhea. She was treated with medications to control her symptoms and given replacement fluids. While they were in the ER, the staff insisted that George receive care as he fell faint. After receiving replacement fluids, he was discharged and found his mother sitting alone in the waiting room with tears running down her face. She was soiled from needing the bathroom. Even though George had asked about her several times, he was told she was fine. When confronted, the staff said they could not do anything else because she had been discharged a few hours before him. They were just following policy. The need for fluids is indisputable and a priority. What could have been done differently to accommodate their unique family situation?

Lee Rite

The vignette is about a man diagnosed with prostate cancer. We will call him Lee Rite. The treatment of choice was external beam radiotherapy. In order to deliver pinpoint rays to very precise areas and limit damage of healthy tissue the patient undergoes a simulation treatment with anatomical marking. In order to record this anatomy, do the marking, and make the body mold one must be 100% unclothed, naked. Lee shared how he felt. The table was cold; the environment was very hard and technical. The young female radiotherapists took measurements and then put red markings on his body to guide therapy. Lee understood what was being done, but felt so frightened, exposed, vulnerable and alone, even though there were two other people in the room. He said he longed for a human connection. He said the staff was as distant and cold as the room and machines.

This procedure took several minutes of positioning, measurement, and marking. Addressing Lee, they always said, Mr. Rite, even though Lee asked them several times to use his first name. This distant clinical approach added to his misery. He asked the radiologist about this stance and was advised, "The staff loose too many patients to have any personal connections." The radiologist implied the staff members are instructed to only use the last name to enhance objective distance and avoid personal involvement to protect themselves.

This was a policy of caring for the staff rather than the patient. And yet, one has to wonder if they had used Lee's first name if it would have changed how he felt. Most likely it was just a symptom and expression of their clinical distance. For many people standing naked before strangers, even professionals, requires some objective distance, even professional distance. While these were strangers, they were health professionals doing a professional practice warranted by their role. Through their education and licensure, society has granted them the right to perform these intimate functions in this therapy setting. The move to protect the staff is an example of how professionals are also human in their response to patients. These practitioners being sterile, cold, and scientific raises a moral issue. This approach communicates fear of involvement when the practitioners could have communicated supportive care. The option was there to transcend one's self or pull back and protect one's self. Caregivers and patients share being human; they are both human persons. There already is a common bond.

John and Lynne

Early June 2013, news agencies across America reported the double suicide of two self-help talk show hosts, John Littig, 48, and Lynne Rosen, 46. John was a motivational speaker and Lynne psychotherapist. CNN reported they led a life-coach consulting agency, "Why Not Now."[86] Their radio talk show, "The Pursuit of Happiness" captured the same theme as expressed in the agency's title. Their self-improvement advice to listeners was optimistic, encouraging listeners to be spontaneous, adventurous, and persevering. Writing an editorial, Amy Anderson in *Culture* (June 6, 2013), focused on the irony of two life coaches who advised, "It's always too early to quit," yet they ended their own lives rather than getting the professional assistance they needed. Anderson focused on the impact of their deaths on the self-help field.

The vulnerabilities of John and Lynne highlight the insufficiency of asserting positive maxims. There needs to be a deeper foundation, a source of inner peace and healing. Notes found with the bodies spoke of Lynne's deep pain, of John's inability to continue in the face of Lynne's pain, and their desire to die together. It seems professional care could have made a difference. For humans, dependence on one's self and self-promotion is just not enough.

---

[86] http://www.life1st.com/files/CPR-Legal_and_Ethical.pdf. CPR Legal and Ethical Issues. 2006.(accessed June 14, 2013)

YouTube footage of the couple during one of their shows featured them advising listeners on a range of tactics for becoming more at ease, including getting "comfortable with change" and doing "something that scares you every day." Thinking is a beautiful thing but so much of life is about impulse. John says emphatically, "Sometimes you just do it!"[87]

The perspective and actions of this couple, John and Lynne, contrasts with the World War II holocaust survivor, Victor Frankl. In *Man's Search for Meaning,* Frankl certainly recommended being in the moment. However he was focused on the present with an eye on an ultimate goal, a reason to live that made today tolerable, even sometimes having desirable moments within the worst of circumstances.

Defiance Makes Vulnerable

On June 18, 2003, the St. Petersburg Newspaper (Florida) carried the story of a ten-year old boy killed by an alligator. One could respond, "Some people just don't pay any attention to the signs not to swim in the ponds." The inland waters in Florida are filled with alligators. Most people wouldn't even walk their dog near a body of water, even a small pond.

The news article had a photograph of green grass and a beautiful blue pond with the tilted ominous white sign, "No swimming. Alligators." The newspaper caption told how his friends pulled him out once, but could do nothing when he disappeared and then surfaced yelling, "Help, help, I don't want to go." That weekend the papers carried the story of the capture and death of four alligators, until they found the 320 pound one that matched the teeth marks on the boy's body.

Laws Protect

So often we want the world to be what we perceive as the way things ought to be. Often college students say that speed limits are made so the state can make money assessing fines. They don't see any reason why one ought to slow for corners if they can maintain control of the car. But that is just the point. A moving object tends toward the direction in which it is going unless opposed by another force; and in a curve an object tends to go straight ahead rather than making the corner. Those who study physics call it centrifugal force. The physicist would draw a curve and an arrow

---

[87] From U tube video of recorded radio program
*www.**youtube**.com/watch?v=MAGym8nPv8w* (accessed on June 10, 2013. No longer available June 22, 2013.)

flying off from the curve in a straight line. Natural forces are real and we must cooperate with them. That is what the engineers have done in the design of airplanes. That is what we do when we reduce our speed and turn into the corner.

The question becomes whether or not there are natural laws, like centrifugal force or the law of gravity, when it comes to the kinds of things humans do. We know that if we consistently overeat we put on weight and if unchecked we get fat. If we tend to tell white lies, not even big ones, or if we tend to take little items from others, not expensive stuff, just little stuff we need, does anything happen to us? Is there anything regular enough to be a law of human nature, like gravity? Can we have the world "our way," or do we have to follow certain rules?

It seems we follow a rule which says, "As something acts, so it is." If you tell lies, then we call you a liar. If you steal, then we call you a thief. Are you? There is another rule young people repeat, "What goes around comes around." So, we can infer there are some stable principles of human action. A study of human life shows that humans have intellects to learn and wills to make choices based on what is known. If you know something you have the truth about it. If you choose to do something you think it is a good thing to do. Even if you choose to break all the rules, at the moment of breaking them, it seemed good to you to break rules and assert your lawlessness, or should I say willfulness. This recalls Aristotle's distinction in the first book of Nicomachean Ethics between the actual good and the apparent good, in other words feeling powerful by breaking civil or laws of nature is only an apparent good. The outcomes can be tragic as with the young boy who swam in the alligator invested pool in Florida.

Codes to Protect Human Rights

The years following World War II with its dramatic violations of human rights, saw the development of international codes: The Nuremburg Codes and The Universal Declaration of Human Rights. The Nuremburg codes emerged from the International Military Tribunal convened in Nuremburg, Germany in 1944 and 1945 to bring to trial 22 German officials. Investigations following the war revealed mass killings and torturing of prisoners in the name of medical science.[88] The Universal Declaration of Human Rights was written by an international committee representing, among others, Canada, France, China, Lebanon, and the

---

[88] http://www.ushmm.org/outreach/en/article.php?ModuleId=10007722(accessed June 10, 2013)

United States. This task force was led by Eleanor Roosevelt. In December 1948, the declarations were adopted by the United Nations General Assembly.[89]

The World Medical Association's congress on human subject's research convening in Helsinki, Finland, 1964, gave rise to the Declarations of Helsinki, Ethical Principles for Medical Research involving Human Subjects. These are thoughtfully amended by the World Medical Association every few years.[90] These human rights were further secured in 1975 (also in Helsinki, Finland) at the first international conference on security and cooperation. Although not a formal treaty, according to the on line Encyclopedia Britannica[91], the Helsinki Accords were an international "agreement (that) recognized the inviolability of the post-World War II frontiers in Europe and pledged the 35 signatory nations to respect human rights and fundamental freedoms and to cooperate in economic, scientific, humanitarian, and other areas."

Human Rights are Patient Rights

As human, the individual has human rights; and, as patient, patient's rights. Most hospitals and health-care facilities post statements of patient's rights. The implementation of these rights depends on the community, culture, and country within which one lives. There are cultural and religious rituals that require us to determine priorities between a religious sanction and human rights or a cultural practice and one's right to humane treatment. In this later, I am thinking of Female Genital Mutilation. This painful and dangerous cutting of young girls is an especially complex occurrence as it is imposed by their own families. To those of us not indoctrinated in the practice, it is unthinkably cruel. But, to those reared with this practice it is a normal rite of passage that is unthinkable to omit. In some cases, young immigrant girls are returned to their country of origin for the procedure as the practice is illegal in the United States and many other countries.[92] When Macklin asserts this mutilation is not exploitation of the powerless because there is no benefit to the more powerful,[93] I disagree as the parents benefit from personal satisfaction and

---

[89] https://en.wikipedia.org/wiki/Universal_Declaration_of_Human_Rights (accessed June 10, 2013)
[90] http://www.wma.net/en/30publications/10policies/b3/ (accessed June 10, 2013)
[91] https://www.britannica.com/event/Helsinki-Accords
[92] https://www.who.int/news-room/fact-sheets/detail/female-genital-mutilation
[93] https://www.unige.ch/medecine/ieh2/files/8714/3472/9172/me-12-Macklin-vulnerability-and-protection.pdf

community status within their culture for having successfully imposed this ritual on their vulnerable daughters.

Laws of Human Nature

The purpose of this discussion of the lawfulness of nature is to consider that there are ways of living that lead to peace and happiness because they are consistent with what it is to be a human being. Alternatively, there are ways of living that lead to chaos and pain because they violate the meaning of life or more simply the natural rules of being human. You can deny the impact of lawless behavior for just so long and then you are nabbed by the 'alligators' of a guilty conscience, anxiety, addiction or disease.

Deep down, at our most thoughtful, humans naturally seek truth and goodness. This tendency leads us to do the good and shun evil. We are happiest when we can look back at the end of the day and see where we have done something beautiful, peaceful, or just. Native Americans and some saintly people, like Saint Francis of Assisi, knew this as they found peace living in harmony with nature. They had no difficulty seeing the lawfulness of nature and the need for humans to conform to natural ways of being.

Being Human as a Foundations of Ethical Standards

Health-care services are delivered within a social system. Achieving government licensure provides warrant to practice as a health-care professional. Scope of practice is generally governed by state licensing boards. The use of specific clinical interventions is guided by discipline specific knowledge. Nonetheless, professional practice is more than these activities. Practitioners interface with individuals in very specific circumstances. The individualistic and personalized nature of health care requires application of principles and modification of environmental settings to meet the health needs of individuals, families, and communities.

All health-care disciplines confront questions of the right or good action so practitioners need to be able to see both clinical and moral principles in a situation. Assistance is given to the moral discernment process through Codes of Ethics established by disciplinary leadership.

Professional Codes

Professional codes as a source for ethical principles were previously addressed. These codes help to specify ethical actions for the practitioner.

However, they are imposed from the outside. Is the good action based on the perspective of a discipline? A physician practicing within the Hippocratic tradition values their liberty to decide what is good for the patient (paternalism) while a more contemporary physician is likely to value patient autonomy. They would explain options and encourage the patient to participate in therapy decisions. This example shows how disciplinary principles can change. Are there any stable norms? We have to seriously consider the potential for stable principles or rules by which one can act and judge actions. In the case of medicine, we have seen principles change based on revised thinking about patient capacity. What if stability were found within moral actions themselves? It is suggested there may be some acts which are good in themselves but one would need a standard or principle by which to judge the action moral.

Law is an External Standard

In addition to professional codes, the law is an external standard for ethical action. To obey the law is the minimum moral standard. Staying within a corporation after learning of illegal or immoral actions by that institution is **implied consent** and makes you subject to the law. To stay within the institution implies agreement with actions done. Setting aside for the moment the question of whether or not abortion is moral, are you supporting abortion when you work for a clinic or hospital that performs the procedure? In another example, during the late 1960's and early 1970's there was much discussion of citizens refusing to have their tax dollars fund the Vietnam War. How closely involved must one be to be accountable for another's action? There is so much uncertainty in the world and so many questions about what corporations are doing. How do you know whether you ought to stay or leave? It is extremely important to know yourself in this regard.

Natural Law Ethics

This section is a short reading on the lawfulness found in nature and human life is taken from a reading of Thomas Aquinas' *Treatise on Laws*.[94] The importance is, if there are standards related to human life, and then there are stable ethical norms unaffected by one's culture or profession.

---

[94] Thomas Aquinas' *Treatise on Laws, Summa Theologicae, questions 90-97.*

Eternal Law

If you accept that there is lawfulness in the universe then there is something meaningful that can be known about being a particular kind of individual, like a bird or a human. This lawfulness can provide ethical standards from the kind of being humans are; from within human life rather than imposed on human actions. By lawfulness in the universe is meant there are some principles like, 2+2 = 4, the meaning of circle, or the Principle of Non-Contradiction (PNC) that are true everywhere and always. They may have been different at some moment but once laid-down with the universe they do not change. They help to define the realities of our world. The PNC says that the same thing cannot both be and not be at the same time in the same respect. Either something is or is not a bird, cat or human. Since equations, geometrical figures, the principles of logic, and definitions of kinds of beings were laid down with the origin of the universe, they do not change. Their particular expressions vary but the laws are eternal. Thomas Aquinas calls this **eternal law.**

The Expression of Eternal Law

The capacity of being able to grow feathers and to fly allows us to recognize a bird. Having a red breast and pulling worms in spring characterizes a robin. Robins pull worms because they are robins. One can recognize a robin by its characteristic behavior but it is not a robin because it pulls worms. The attribute (characteristic behavior) flows from being a robin.

What are the defining characteristics of a human? The defining characteristics of human nature are the expression of the eternal within humanity. These defining characteristics are uniquely human, normal for humans to have but not shared with other non-human things. Within the Aristotelian-Thomistic tradition these are the intellect and will, the ability to reason with immaterial concepts and freedom of choice based on this knowledge. Notice that this is not just problem solving. Other animals can problem-solve, but they cannot contemplate the meaning of life or what it is to have family or knowledge. Some animals care about their family unit, but they don't concern themselves with what it means to have family. Immaterial concepts are separated from matter and particular circumstances, like the meaning of the term "tree" or the meaning of yellow roses expressing friendship. Intellectual capacities allow humans to seek truth and to debate about "what truth is." Because of the potential for knowledge, humans have choices, options. It is characteristic of humans to have intellect and will, to seek truth and to choose the good. As human we have the freedom to choose evil, but the positive or actual choice is the good. Even when one chooses evil they do it thinking their action will bring something desirable or good. Truth and good ness are the eternal within human nature. The defining characteristics of human nature are the expression of the eternal within human.

The Expression of the Eternal within Human Life is Natural Law

Human nature is that which unites all humans as human (the same kind of existent being) and is characterized as having knowledge and choice. These capacities are directly related to accountability in moral action. It may seem repetitive, but it is important to recall a moral action is freely chosen based on knowledge of circumstances and knowledge of principles that apply in those particular circumstances. The moral or proper action is freely chosen as the good to be done in the situation. That situations and individuals involved vary is sometimes taken to mean that there are no stable moral norms. However, the view we are discussing would hold that principles remain stable within changing circumstances. This is part of the interest and challenge of human life. So often when we want to do something, we say that the principle does not apply to us or the circumstance of the rule is different. Excuses we hear might include: "I'm not that diabetic;" "They aren't truly married;" "The particular circumstance doesn't fit;" "This pie isn't that sweet;" or "What happened wasn't sex." Our moral responsibility for what we have chosen to do is based on what we know, unless we have chosen to be ignorant.

Natural Law Ethics Guides Human Life

This capacity to pursue truth and choose the good is foundational to Natural Law Ethics. This position holds that what it is to be human is within human nature laid down with the universe and thus participating in Eternal Law. The first principle of Natural Law Ethics is also the first principle of practical reason: "Do good; avoid evil." There are three rules that follow: (1) preserve human life; (2) educate the young; and (3) live in peace. These precepts of Natural Law are philosophically derived from what it is to be human because pursuing truth and goodness requires that one be alive, educated, and living in peace. These are not rules imposed externally. They are within the human as actor. Additionally, these rules are known on the basis of reason rather than faith. They provide stable norms for human action outside of a specific culture, religion, or profession. In fact, a professional position can be evaluated by these standards. They tell us the transition in medical ethics to valuing patient autonomy honors the human capacity for knowledge and choice. These natural standards lead to the conclusion that the patient must be provided sufficient information to make a reasonable choice.

Human Law

Having free will, humans have the potential for good and evil. In order to live in ordered communities, individuals must follow the laws developed by their government. **Human laws** are developed as standards for a peaceful ordered existence in society. Most human laws preserve Natural Law and thus, Eternal Law. Human laws that preserve Natural Law are just and lead to a just society. Examples of these laws include promoting education of the young, stopping at intersections, protection of property, and equal opportunity for employment.

Divine Law

Because humans often make unjust laws and because we cannot judge a person's intent, Aquinas held that it is necessary to have a fourth kind of law. These laws are provided by the designer of the universe who laid down the eternal laws and are called **Divine Law**. They prepare one for an eternal existence with the divine origin of the universe.

Awareness of the standards of Natural Law was behind the international standards promoted in the "United Nations Universal Declaration of Human Rights." Jacques Maritain, a famous Thomistic scholar, played a leading role in the drafting committee.[95]

Conclusion

This chapter ends with a reflection, entitled "Why…?" written for an informal employee newsletter from 1985. I was working as a visiting nurse, and the reflection on the experience answered the question whether severely disabled individuals ought to be at home.

One Friday afternoon, I telephoned the home of an elderly paralyzed patient to arrange the next day's visit. I spoke to her grandson, who said that he usually cared for her and would be home. We agreed upon a time.

---

[95] www.firstthings.com/article/2007/01/**maritains**-true-humanism--7 (accessed June 22, 2013)

It was a bright and sunny Saturday afternoon, I drove into an older section of town where many homes needed repair and front doors stood sagging ajar. But, for some reason, the roses and daisies always seemed more beautiful in these yards. The street where my patient lived was just past "Baby Dee's Private Club." Driving down the street, I became acutely aware of the stares of a group of men standing by a fence on the side of the road. Upon reaching the corner, I realized with a heavy sigh that I had apparently passed the house because the numbers were beyond my destination. Since I was driving a Volkswagen Beetle, the intersection was plenty large enough to make the turn back. Trying to ignore the men, I stopped my car before an unmarked house across from where they were standing. Considering if it could be the right house, I looked up to see, a rough-looking young man, wearing only faded jeans unbuckled at the waist, sauntering towards my car. I rolled the window down a little in response to his tapping. "You lookin' for Miss...?" he drawled. As the faint odor of alcohol filled my car, I answered "yes." "This is the house," he continued, "I talked to you yesterday." Somewhat relieved, but uneasy, I got out of the car and followed him into the house.

Once inside, he coarsely proclaimed our arrival to a lady upstairs and hurried toward the center hall. In a small bulge next to the stairwell were crowded a hospital bed, TV, and rugged end table. The elderly heavy-set lady was lying on her side toward the noisy TV. The young man explained that his grandmother was unable to speak or move, but that she knew we were there and that she liked him to sit and watch TV with her. He turned and said a few words to her. His face softened and love shown from his eyes. During the examination, it became apparent that her under pad was soiled. I assisted him to wash her and change the pad. As he turned to care for his mute and helpless grandmother, his gentleness and respect touched my heart—they expressed a tenderness and love rarely seen.

This helpless, mute, semi-alert grandmother, seemingly more dead than alive, was giving what might be the greatest gift a person can give. She was giving her rough street-wise boy an opportunity to know love and the gift of giving love. This tenderness may not have occurred in any other circumstance.

Remembering this account for you, still brought vivid memories and a full heart, I am acutely aware our world is dearly in need of such love. If you have the opportunity to love or to allow someone to love you, let the tenderness and power of that love warm your heart and dispel the chill of winter, the grief of loss, and the anxiety of our uncertain future. It seems I am asking a lot of love, but I don't think so. Love is the greatest gift we can give or receive. It is a most powerful force for peace. Let me conclude with the few lines used to conclude this little story when it was first written. "Love is a gentle gift; a gift that gives—not only to the one loved, but to the one who love.

Conversation Starters:
1. Describe two experiences you have had as a sales clerk or customer or in health care. For one of these describe an experience that left you emotionally flat or drained of energy and one that left you stronger or happier and more peaceful. After preparing these describe how they were the same and how different. Can you identify what made the enriching experience richer, happier and more peaceful?
2. List five things you can do to increase the positive impact on those who come within your area of influence. This may include work, school, or family.
3. Seedhouse, in his discussion in Chapter Five, thought it was possible to communicate human caring without becoming attached. What do you think? How could the isolation of Mr. Rite have been bridged without becoming sensual?
4. Describe what you would do if you saw a conflict between hospital policy and one of the standards of human rights?

Reflection Submissions:
1. Describe your reaction to the suggestion that you have a moral obligation to have a positive impact on those you encounter. Provide your reasoned argument for or against this obligation. A reasoned argument asserts your position and good reasons to accept this position.
2. Obtain a copy of your disciplinary code of ethics. Write a short paper of how your codes are similar and different from the Universal Declaration of Human Rights, and either the Nuremburg Codes or the Helsinki Accords.
3. Write a one to two-page historical summary of the development of one of these sets of standards: Universal Declaration of Human Rights, Nuremburg Codes, or the Helsinki Accords (or Declarations).

Outline for Chapter 6: The Patient is also a Person
A. The Patient is First a Human Being
B. Vulnerability
    1. Vulnerability follows injury and illness
    2. Vulnerability due to limited freedom
    3. Caregiver vulnerability
    4. Financial and educational vulnerabilities

Terminology for Chapter 6
Implied consent
Eternal Law
Natural Law
Human Law
Divine Law
Person
Vulnerable
Conscientious objection
Rights and responsibilities

SECTION FOUR:

ETHICAL REASONING AND ETHICAL THEORIES

The early sections of this book developed a philosophical understanding of being human and our need for community, be that a small, intimate union or society at large. We are natural substances with capacities beyond nature for knowing and choosing, that is making choices based on knowledge of universal principles and particular circumstances.

We are now concerned with clear careful ethical reasoning and statements that can serve as guiding principles in the practical syllogism. Chapter Seven is "The Right Action Requires Discernment and Virtue," a discussion of virtue ethics and ethical decision making. Chapter Eight, "A Short Overview of Philosophical Ethical Perspectives," provides a review of several ethical theories that can guide personal ethical decisions. All of this work of reason is prior to action. It is reflective. Once a decision is made, the move to action requires good judgment and courage to act or not act as indicated by reason.

CHAPTER 7

THE RIGHT ACTION REQUIRES DISCERNMENT AND VIRTUE

Objectives

This chapter provides an opportunity for you to:

1. Describe virtue and the need for virtue in the moral life.
2. Compare Aristotle's six kinds of persons in living a moral life.
3. Discern the human good in particular situations.
4. Compare your decision making with that recommended by Plato, Aristotle, and Augustine.
5. Develop ethical decision-making capacity.

The Need for Virtue

In Chapter Three, we noted that nature acts generally and for the most part. Scientific generalizations from research have an element of uncertainty until one has insight into clear relationships and can reason with confidence that "If and only if the antecedent, then the consequence occurs (**Iff** p, then q)." Recall the work of William Harvey, we discussed that the blood can be proven to return to the heart in a closed system with limited volume, if and only if there are small vessels at the extremity of blood flow (now known as capillaries).

Knowledge of causal relationships on the supposition of the end was also considered. There are days and days of sunny rain and no rainbow, but if there is a rainbow there must be rain, sun, and the proper angle between the raindrop and the eye of the observer.

Human actions are the most uncertain in all of nature because of our freedom. We often know what ought to be done and then do something completely different or nothing. Plato was convinced that if a person really knew what ought to be done, they would do it. This would be the action that participated in the ultimate Form of Good. Knowledge of the Good and identifying this Good in the current situation would compel us to act well, to perform right actions.[96]

As was said earlier, Aristotle disagreed with Plato that one would do the good if it were known because very often we know what ought to be done and do not do it.[97] Aristotle separated decisions from knowledge and action. He believed acting well was more complex than just knowing what ought to be done. He taught "choice" was not made with a decision of the best act but at the moment of action,[98] additionally, what is actually done reflects who one is, rather than just one's knowledge. Knowledge of principles, the given situation, and the prudential judgment that this is a case of a moral principle are necessary for right action but not sufficient. Right action also requires a habit of acting well (virtue), especially the virtue of courage. When faced with a desired object and experiencing desire or appetite or especially lust, anger or fear, strong emotion can overturn reason. The principle is still known but reason clouds over and it is only known like an actor reciting lines. To stay with what ought to be done, one needs practice in following knowledge rather than appetite. After appetite is satisfied, or the anger or fear dissipates clear thinking returns and remorse sets in if one has acted outside their moral norms

The Four Cardinal Virtues

Within classical virtue theory, virtue is required to even see the good end as a good to be achieved,[99] be that end education or a good reputation or keeping one's word. Virtue is also essential to keep emotions in check and to focus on the decision one has made. While reading this, you may be thinking, virtue is self-discipline and you would be right. This self-discipline is the virtue of **Moderation**. Right action also requires good judgment or **Wisdom** in order to know what ought to be done, and **Courage** to act on the known proper behaviors. **Justice** and moderation are principles of action: moderation in the control of one's appetites and justice or fairness in how we treat others. Without self-control we cannot achieve inner peace or justice. Virtue ethics is grounded in personal development. Virtue requires childhood training, formation, and then it can be strengthened by one's moral choices. The virtue ethicist would say to act in the way you want to be. Today's actions are making who you will

---

[96] Developed from Plato, *Republic* VI and VII

[97] *Nicomachean Ethics (NE)*, Translated with an Introduction by Martin Ostwald, Indianapolis, Indiana: The Liberal Arts Press, Inc. 1962. Book VII, 4.

[98] *NE*, VI, 2.

[99] *NE*, II

be tomorrow. In some sense, the goal of virtue ethics is inner harmony, the philosopher's definition of happiness,[100] ideally, this inner peace overflows into peace in the community. Virtues are human excellences and allow for the best in human living. A peaceful family, organization or community emerges from peace within individual members. The law, policies, and rules can only impose order. These measures go a long way towards bringing peace, but they are not enough.

Six Characteristic Human Responses

Probably not for judging individuals, but for understanding humanity, Aristotle identified six characteristic responses to situations requiring a moral choice[101] these responses place humans on a continuum. The least capable he calls a (1) **brute,** someone incapable of knowing and doing the moral action because of mental limitations. This person functions best when told what to do. He then identifies the (2) **vicious** or evil person who rationalizes everything done. In his or her mind, they have never done anything wrong. They have reasons for doing everything they want to do. People within this designation are self-indulgent. They believe they ought to pursue whatever they desire and their reason supports their efforts. Since they never see themselves as doing anything wrong, they never have moral conflict or remorse. They never say "I'm sorry." The (3) **weak-willed person** has knowledge of moral principles and can reason what ought to be done, but at the last minute does what is desired, not what is known as the best action to be done. After desire is satisfied, sorrow and remorse flood the soul. Weak-willed persons wish they had been strong enough to do the known good action. They promise they will be different, next time, but usually this does not happen. The (4) **strong-willed person** also has knowledge of principles and reasons clearly to what ought to be done. The difference is this person usually does the intended good action. The strong-willed person has a habit of following through with what they reason ought to be done. Both the weak-willed and strong-willed person experience moral conflict and then remorse if desire is fulfilled and the good can no longer be done. One can shrug their shoulders and say, "Don't cry over spilt milk," or "You can't fix broken eggs." Nonetheless, the failure does deserve notice and correction. This undesirable action will make future unwanted behaviors easier to perform.

Many years ago, during a time of presidential and television evangelist

---

[100] *NE*, VII, 3.
[101] *NE*, VII.

scandals, a radio speaker said something similar to "First comes the failure, then the fall, but with the fall comes the fall out. The key is to avoid the failures, the small indiscretions." Aristotle would say to avoid situations of your personal vulnerabilities. This may seem crude but he would say, "Don't go into the bedroom unless you plan to use the bed." Don't set yourself up for failure or misunderstanding. If you're tempted to drink heavily, don't go into the bar or an alcohol indulgent party. In fact, he held that a person who performs a crime under the influence of alcohol ought to pay double penalty because he chose to cloud reason, the first crime.[102]

To do the good that ought to be done while confronting appetite, fear, and hunger requires the four cardinal virtues addressed earlier. These are good judgment (also called wisdom or prudence) to know what is right, courage to act contrary to how one feels, moderation for self-control, and justice in care of others, but especially courage. Aristotle was especially interested to explain how individuals can know what to do and not do it. He was thinking of us all, but first, there are two additional types of persons, to be described. The (5) **naturally moral person** is inclined by nature to see and do what ought to be done in all situations. In order to explain this, Aristotle suggested this person is subjected to weak appetites and passions, so reason stays in control. In contrast to the evil person, who always sees it as right to do what he or she desires, this naturally moral person's appetite quickly follows reason. The final characterization is the (6) **ideal individual** with all moral capacity of the naturally moral person, but also with an attractive appearance, ideal family, political system, education, ideal upbringing, and opportunities. This ideal individual cannot exist, but is the positive opposite of the natural brute without moral capacity, and stands as the goal or end to be sought in human life.

To See the Good and Do the Good

If one would be a happy, virtuous person, then one needs to see the good as that which ought to be done; then use good judgment to determine the action that leads to this perceived goodness. One needs to do the known good even in small things. This is motivation to not cheat or steal even in little things. Recall, even nature only acts generally and for the most part. One can do all of these things and still fall into a moral lapse. Reasoning on the supposition of the end, if we meet someone who is a happy moral person, someone we can truly admire, we can be sure their

---

[102] *NE*, VII, 1145b 9-10.

upbringing brought them capacities to control appetite and treat others with respect. They have been particular but not slavish to follow expected standards. One does not act with virtue by accident.

Ironically, as this is being written, I am sitting in a restaurant, using their electricity to power my notebook. I commented to the young lady cleaning tables about using their electricity, and I hoped it was acceptable. She said it was alright because teenagers sit here all the time recharging their cell phones. One can rationalize that they paid for a meal and their presence encourages business, but something is wrong. Actually, I asked the wrong person. Management sets the rules. Even so, what another is doing is not a good standard; even if "everyone is doing it," as a teen argues to his or her mother. This consideration of what others are doing is an external review that makes the community standard the moral norm, which may or may not lead to the right actions. Aristotle wanted a standard based on the meaning of being a virtuous person and what the virtuous person would do.

A Virtuous Action

A virtuous action requires that an individual act intentionally, that is purposefully. One must have knowledge of the situation and that an action is required, as well as options. The action must be chosen, and it must spring from a stable character of virtuous actions. This requirement of knowledge and being freely chosen is part of the consideration of responsibility for one's actions. In being virtuous one must avoid extreme behaviors. Virtue is destroyed by deficiency and excess, pain and pleasure. Aristotle writes,

> I am referring to moral virtue: for it is moral virtue that is concerned with emotions and actions, and it is in emotions and actions that excess, deficiency, and the median are found. Thus we can experience fear, confidence, desire, anger, pity, and generally any kind of pleasure and pain either too much or too little, and in either case not properly. But to experience all this at the right time, toward the right objects, toward the right people, for the right reason, and in the right manner – that is the median and the best course, the course that is a mark of virtue. …We may thus conclude that virtue or excellence is a characteristic involving choice, and that it consists in observing the mean relative to us, a mean which is defined by a rational principle, such as a man of practical wisdom would use to determine it. It is the mean by reference to two vices: the one of excess and the other of deficiency…Hence, in respect of its essence and the definition of its essential nature virtue is a mean, but in regard to

goodness and excellence it is an extreme.[103]

Finding the Median

The following are a summary of Aristotle's instructions for finding the median: 1) obtain knowledge of the situation; 2) identify and avoid extremes; 3) seek counsel of those respected as virtuous and knowledgeable in the content area in which one must decide; 4) be aware of your tendencies to excess and deficiency, and choose away from them. He adds:

We must watch the errors which have the greatest attraction for us personally. For the natural inclination of one man (person) differs from that of another, and we each come to recognize our own (inclinations) by observing the pleasure and the pain produced in us (by the different extremes). We must then draw ourselves away in the opposite direction, for by pulling away from error we shall reach the middle (parenthetical content added)[104]

A Role Model

Aristotle recognizes that virtue ethics requires a role model, a guide in one's initial development and counsel when facing difficult decisions. It is encouraging that a person who recognizes their lack of moral awareness or decision-making capacity can turn to a trained guide or counselor. Within Greek culture proper conduct is recognized by the praise and blame of the community. Historically and personally we have seen that majority view can be wrong and leads away from virtue. This is likely why Aristotle spends much time on inner attributes of virtue. This requirement of a role model is a difficulty with virtue ethics; one needs a way of evaluating the role model.

Human Excellence

Virtue, as a human excellence, presumes humans can act in ways that are excellent. It presumes that humans can be improved, even perfected. What evidence is there that human conduct can be improved? What would this mean, anyway? What makes one think we can evaluate human excellence? What would human excellence mean? To answer these questions, one would need to consider how humans are different from

---

[103] *NE*, II, 6.
[104] *NE*, II, 9.

other beings in the world. Earlier, we said humans are different in their capacity to have knowledge of concepts and to reason on this conceptual level. Another way humans are different, radically different, is that we are free to determine many aspects of our own lives. We called this free will. Human excellence and the human good must be related to these capacities of knowledge and freedom.

The Human Good

How can one argue human good exists when we experience so much evil? It is very clear evil exists, especially when listening to or reading the news, but what kind of existence does the good or goodness have? If a moral action is a principle-based action towards the human good, we need to know what the phrase means, "towards the human good." What is the term "good" a sign of and what is the term pointing to? In the preceding chapter we explored that human excellence or goodness is concerned with knowledge and freedom as these are unique human attributes, but we did not challenge the term "good." Is "good" an attribute, like a good student, a state of being to be achieved, like good health, or something in itself, like Plato's Form of the Good? Preceding chapters referred to Plato, for whom The Good was highest perfection in a place of perfections, and the origin and sustainer of all that exists. Plato's Good also makes knowledge possible as existent items are recognized in the world around us. From a Platonic understanding, what one ought to do becomes clear as one draws near to Beauty, Truth, and Unity, the transcendentals identified with the ultimate Good. Choosing and doing the moral action preserves these transcendentals, and thus goodness.[105]

If goodness is not an existent state of perfection (The Good) in a world of perfection, could it be a state of being, or an attribute that can be found in the world around us as Aristotle held? In the *Nicomachean Ethics,* Aristotle rejects Plato's understanding of goodness as The Good. The term "good" is used in so many ways, it could not be just one thing.[106] We use the term to apply to a good pen, a good meal, a good day, a good person, a good book. If there is a common meaning in "good," perhaps "good" means the item is the fullness of what it ought to be. The pen writes smoothly, the meal is satisfying in variety and amount, the day brought work and pleasure, etc. This understanding of good as variable according

---

[105] S. E. Stumpf, *Philosophy: History & Problems, 5th ed. New York: McGraw Hill, 1994, pp. 46-69.*
[106] *NE*, I, 6.

to the item is the reason Aristotle proposed the ideal moral person could be the standard of goodness for which humans strive. We are left to ask how moral goodness is acquired. What evidence is there that humans can improve or even be good? Aristotle would hold that, at least, we can be good some times because we keep expecting it. Think of the number of times we exhort people to do what we think is good or right: "Be kind," "You need to share," "You need to lose weight." According to Aristotle, we would not keep providing this advice if it had no effect. We may not agree on what is the good, but we seek it. We agree some behaviors bring more peace, or knowledge, or emotional and physical well-being. Different people propose different behaviors to gain this peace, but the search is common to all humans.

Augustine

The early fifth century scholar, Augustine struggled to understand how there could be both an infinite good and evil in the world. Augustine, early in his life, argued that if there were an infinite good, there would be no room for evil. Being infinite means being everywhere and always. If this were true, he reasoned, the good would leave no room for evil. Evil is obvious, as experienced in all of our lives. So for many years Augustine denied the existence of an infinite good. In his important book, *On Free Choice of the Will*,[107] written after his acceptance of Platonic philosophy and Christianity, Augustine explains evil as the absence of the good or goodness. It has no positive existence of its own. Within natural disasters there is a lack of order and proportion which are the goods in natural design. In illness, there is a loss of physical integrity. Additionally, what seems disordered to us may be ordered within a more universal perspective. Human evil is chosen by individuals thinking it is good. Human freedom is seen as precious. Augustine came to accept Plato's understanding of the universe as having its origin in an ultimate Good. This insight led him to give up his skepticism and accept the existence of a creator, sustainer God. For Augustine, this Creator values human freedom so much that He allows moral evil rather than interfere with human freedom. He also teaches that we, humans are in conformity with goodness when the right things are loved. When confronted with a situation, a decision can be made by considering what value is reflected in each possible decision. He thought human excellence was achieved by ordering

---

[107] Augustine, Bk. I, Trans. A.S. Benjamin or E.J. Hackstaff. Indianapolis, Indiana: Hackett Publishing Company, Inc. 1993.

what we love from the material to the immaterial and preferring the higher immaterial goods.[108] Faced with the decision of whether to go to the party or study, one would have greater excellence in choosing to study. Not that there is anything wrong with going to a party, but for Augustine to gain knowledge is a higher good than pleasure. Knowledge is immaterial concepts, while pleasure is associated with the body. Of course, you may be going to the party for the sake of friendship, which is an immaterial universal concept, like the truths one can come to know. Given this example, we see friendship places the party at a higher level than going because it is fun. Augustine's ranking would depend on why you are going.

Aristotle

Aristotle would probably tell you go to the party, but don't stay too long because you also need to complete your studies. Aristotle thought excellence was in having moderation or balance in one's life. Let this suffice for showing differences in finding excellence or goodness. An action may have goodness in different ways: 1) the action may have its goodness in the action itself, like the simple joy of going to a movie with a friend; 2) the good might be in the outcome but not the action itself, like going to the doctor or dentist or training for a future event when you do not like the training; 3) the good might both be in the action and its outcome. An example of this later is an athlete who enjoys training, as well as the good outcome of gaining strength. Virtue is good in itself for its immediate result in the active situation, but it is also good in its impact bringing the actor virtue and inner peace.[109]

Ethical Decision Making

The above discussions of virtue and finding the human good have been for further development of decision-making capacity by practicing moral reasoning. Having a good grasp of practical decision-making will provide helpful guidance when facing moral difficulties and ethical dilemmas in the clinical setting. The basic practical syllogism described earlier was an argument with two premises. The first premise is a principle, policy or rule stating what ought to be done, i.e. "One must not steal." The second premise is the particular circumstance(s) with which one is confronted. For

---

[108] Stumpf, pp.144-47.
[109] *NE*, I.

the sake of our discussion, this would be sitting in a fast food restaurant that does not invite computer users using their electricity. The conclusion is whether or not the situation is a case of the rule. Is this usage of electricity stealing? Does this moral maxim apply to my situation? Am I bound by the rule to not steal? I am well aware that moral errors occur by not seeing that the rule or principle applies to the actor or that the situation does not meet the requirements of the rule, when it does. Am I costing the restaurant money? Am I taking what is not mine? Honesty is one of my core values, so I spoke with the manager and was given permission to use the electricity. I was very happy the manager understood my concern and did not think my request trivial.

In class one evening, when we were discussing where to draw the line for stealing, we noted that most students would never take an office computer, but they often take pens, paper clips and printer paper. Students often do work on "company time" and while the most sincere religious persons would never steal, they have no problem photocopying personal items or material for a church function while at work. During this discussion, the following anonymous story was told. A young girl was preparing posters for school. She had brought home poster paper, markers and paste. Her father comes home and with surprise asks, "Where did you get all these supplies." The girl answers, "From school." Her father loudly proclaims, "I told you not to take stuff from school. Just ask, and I will bring it from the office."

How does one discern fair use? We must avoid becoming frozen by fear we are stealing, but must also respect the property of others and cannot be blind to our behavior when we take what is not ours. What would be a reasonable middle ground?

Reflection Grows Ethical Capacity

We found earlier that ethical actions are principle based actions toward the human good. We considered sources of principles in professional codes, institutional policies, and statements of human rights. The laws in your community reflect the least you are expected to do as a member of that community. They are important to consider as minimum moral standards for all persons. "You can at least obey the law." In addition to laws, health professionals are expected to at least, "Do no harm." Philosophically we have considered ethical support of principles or maxims from within the kind of being involved in moral action, i.e. humans, and the requirements of practice, which call the practitioner to be responsible to care because of the patient's vulnerability.

At this point, we turn to the process of ethical reasoning and the development of decision-making capacity. The goal is to take the mystery out of listening and thinking when confronted with ethical dilemmas so that you may act in a way true to yourself and your chosen profession, that is, with integrity. Although you may feel pressured, you do not want to rush into a decision, you need to take the time to gather information, ask questions and think out your decision. Having a set of questions, a process of reasoning will enable you to resolve the situation into an appropriate action. Problem is, often there is no such time. The situation is confronting and needs a prompt response. Because of this, it is important to come apart from the clinical setting to discuss and reflect on moral concerns and decisions that have been made and need to be made. When you have acted on a difficult decision you would benefit from taking a bit of time to think about what happened. Reflection will enable you to grow in ethical capacity. While doing this, remember that you made the best decision you could with the information and time you had.

Practical Syllogism

Until now, we have only used the practical syllogism but there are additional models or formats of moral reasoning. To review, the practical syllogism is found in personal moral decisions based on known principles of interpersonal actions applied in particular circumstances resulting in the conclusion that this is a case of the known principle, i.e. First premise: "It's wrong to steal, and it's wrong to lie;" Second premise: cheating on this exam involves stealing someone else's work and lying to the teacher by presenting it as my own; Conclusion: therefore, I cannot copy the answers. The second premise in this example already jumps beyond description to an intermediate conclusion which leads to the action conclusion that, "I cannot copy the answers." There is an application of principle in this particular situation, because this situation is a case of the principle, "It is wrong to steal and lie."

Analogical Reasoning

Moral reasoning may also resolve an ethical dilemma by seeing the similarities between this situation and a legal precedent, a landmark case that serves as a model for similar action. Recall our discussion of the ground-breaking Karen Ann Quinlan case that has been a pattern for the removal of ventilators for many health care professionals and families for more than thirty years. To use this **analogical reasoning**, one has to assess the significant similarities and differences between the historic case and the current situation. A match becomes a significant argument for doing the same thing that was done in the past.

Ethical Analysis

The intent is not to provide an exhaustive list of moral reasoning, but a guide, a way of proceeding. When confronting a situation with moral tension, if there is not a match between principle and situation, and there is not a legal precedent, one may be facing an ethical dilemma that requires exposition of the situation with identification of the personal and professional values and principles that are in conflict. One begins by gathering needed knowledge: interpersonal, clinical, ethical, and legal. There needs to be identification of the primary decision-maker and the options open to you if you are not the primary decision-maker. One would consider what ought to be done given these intellectual and practice factors. Before you act, though, you must imaginatively check the positive and negative impact of your action on the persons and institutions involved. You will probably want to take actions that will provide the greatest benefit or reduce negative impacts. Taking the time to envision outcomes and factoring these into the decision does not mean one is using consequentialist ethics. All decision-makers whatever one's theoretical preference need to consider consequences of one's actions. A **consequentialist position** gives priority to outcomes and exclusively considers outcomes valuable. Our discussion of various ethical positions continues in the next chapter.

Signs you are confronting an ethical dilemma where you will need to use your practical reasoning and analysis include: experiencing tension and high energy, there are strong emotions experienced in yourself and others, there is often a question of life and death. Questions of right and wrong lead to conflicting options and often strongly held positions are behind experienced conflict. When principles conflict and there are good reasons for doing different things you will experience moral tension. If the situation is such that once an action is taken you cannot go back and take the other option, you are within an **ethical dilemma**. An ethical dilemma is a situation where a decision must be made. There are good reasons for doing two different things, and once an action is taken you cannot go back and do the other option. The situation is even more difficult when the contextual pressure does not lend itself to reflection; and hesitancy could cost a life.

Confronting Ethical Dilemmas

When confronting an ethical dilemma you need to listen carefully, think clearly, and act with integrity.

Listen Carefully

Listen to Inner Self

This is the voice of your past. It will tell you about your values, your emotions, impulses and your fears. (The threat you may feel in the situation.) Ask yourself, what is the middle ground between impulsive action and no action? What would you want people to remember you did in the situation? This is a good moment to consider the assessment tools given by Tom Michaud in *The Virtue of Business Ethics*.[15] He purposed a simple assessment based on virtue ethics. The ethical action is found by looking for the Honorable (how you would want to be known), the Beneficial (the long term good for the community as a whole) and the Legal (this includes the law, policies, and codes).

Listen to the Situation

What calls out to be done? There will be some things that seem immediate, but on a further deeper inquiry there may be another action that would be more helpful. You need to ask a lot of questions and look for this long term good, the Beneficial.

Listen to the Law, Codes, and Policies

All three of these are usefully captured by Michaud as the Legal. Earlier we discussed and had activity questions related to professional codes and institutional policies, which are applied statements of what is legal in your country, state, county, and institution. We have also considered what is due a person just because they are human (United Nations and Nuremberg codes of Human Rights). These codes and policies guide and support decisions that you make as a professional. The law is especially important in what it prevents or prohibits. You will recall that what is permitted in law is minimal moral standard for the entire community. When a law is violated, you have gone beyond or did not uphold what is accepted by your community.

Listen to Sources of Ethical Principles

These sources are humanity, parents, society, school, and church. Those who study classical philosophy and moral action hold that it means something to be human. Humanity is unique in the world. We are the living being that can reason and have choices based on knowledge. Natural Law Ethics holds this capacity to reason and choose provides a foundation for, preserving life, educating the young, and living in peace. If humans have the capacity to know, that is, to seek the truth one has to be alive and educated to do so. If humans have the capacity of choice, we need to choose well. In order to do that you need to be alive and to have experienced goodness. You also need the emotional distance that will allow you to think. This is where living in peace enters the picture.

Society, school and church doctrines help to form our choices. They help us understand right and wrong so we can choose well. There are a variety of social and religious principles. Having these principles as a part of your life allows you to usually make decisions by simply matching principles and situations, thus avoiding ethical dilemmas unless there is a conflict of principles.

In summary, an ethical dilemma calls one to listen: Listen to yourself (your values), to the ethical codes of your profession, the policy manual of your institution, and the law. Listen to sources of ethical principles: humanity, society, church. Listen to the perspectives of others involved in the situation. Careful listening concludes with (1) a statement of the apparent ethical dilemma and (2) identification of relevant ethical content in the situation, codes, principles and awareness of your perspective, and that of other persons involved. More important even than the statement of dilemma are the questions that emerge. Listening provides content for reflection. Your thinking will be flawed and your decisions faulty if you do not have all of the information or if you do not take the time to think through the situation. When caught in an ethical dilemma, you never stop listening. You need to stay open to new information and changes in the situation. Very often the dilemma dissolves with clear understanding of what is happening and involved parties gain important information and insights. This is especially true with end of life decisions. It takes time and thoughtful communications for family members to grasp the patient's state of being and what can be hoped for.

Think Clearly

In order to think clearly you need to get some emotional distance. Strong emotion clouds reason, as we noted above. Identify relevant content, values, and principles in this situation. The emphasis is on "this." It is important to separate this situation from your personal opinions and past experiences. Identify the primary decision maker. Very often we get involved in clinical discussions and reflections about situations as if the decision were ours when it is not. Even though the decision is not yours, you need to consider relevant principles and facts of the case to decide if you are able to be a part of decisions and actions which are taken. You need to respect your education and your conscience positions. If you perceive what is happening as immoral you need to express your views, maybe even to excuse yourself from the setting. Your positions expressed need to be well founded, not just emotional. As the conclusion of your thoughtful analysis your views may be very helpful to others in your health-care team and the decision makers. With expressing your views, though, it is very important to follow institutional policies. You will likely not be at liberty to speak as you might wish to with patients and families, but you do need to have trusted staff members with whom you can discuss the situation.

If you decide to act, you need to check the impact of your actions on all parties involved. While you were listening, you were already thinking. This allowed you to hear the ethical dilemma and select ethically relevant content. In fact, you may have jumped to a conclusion that made you irritated or concerned. You may have felt like your "head was spinning" with ideas. These need to be sorted out and unrealistic options discarded.

Be assured that if you had to make an immediate decision, you probably did the very best you could with the information you had to resolve the situation with which you were confronted. One of the advantages of taking a course in ethics is to take the time to step back and look at the process of decision making and the decisions made.

Most learning in ethical reasoning comes with reflection on what happened in previous situations. Every time you step back and reflect on your decisions you grow in self-understanding and the ability to listen and think more clearly in the future. You have made a good start in developing ethical reasoning. We will consider a few more important abilities as we focus on sorting options while seeking to resolve dilemmas.

Sorting Options as a Way of Thinking

Sorting options to determine what ought to be done includes (1) seeing through the situation to a principle that applies in the situation. Acceptance of a principle guides what one ought to do in the situation. (2) Identifying similar cases and the way they were resolved will assist in thinking analogically about the present situation. Cases resolved in the courts are very important; even if you're not sure similar cases ought to lead to the same decision. (3) When different principles and codes apply in a situation advising different actions, one must establish priorities among the principles. For example, when faced with the apparent need to lie to save someone's life. There is a clash between truth-telling and valuing life.

Some hold life is a higher value; others hold "one must tell the truth at all costs." This is a good time to look for a middle-ground solution. A Jehovah's Witness friend shared that during World War II, when the Nazi soldiers were searching for Jews being sheltered in homes, Witnesses deflected the question, "Do you have Jews hidden in your house?" They would answer, "Look and see." They reasoned that soldiers were going to search anyway and they were sure the so called fugitives were well hidden. (4) An important capacity in resolving an ethical dilemma is the ability to identify the extreme options, i.e., doing nothing or doing everything. Once the extremes are available, it is easier to see the middle ground. While this sorting is helpful in all perspectives, virtue ethics holds that the middle or moderate action is close to or actually the moral action.

We have previously acknowledged the importance of practical reason making a match between a situation and the principle that applied in the situation and reasoning analogically to match this situation with a similar classical case. In this section we have also considered the important abilities of establishing a priority of principles and seeking a compromise or middle position between extremes. All of these activities of practical reasoning presume the ability to see the moral action as desirable, the ability to make good decisions and the inner strength to actually act on the decision made. This insight and these abilities or virtues were discussed earlier. Habits of acting well, virtues, are almost essential to making one's own ethical decisions. If one does not have a habit of acting with justice and integrity, it is essential to follow the advice of others who do have the training and education to make good decisions in difficult situations. With practice you can develop the habit of good judgment yourself.

Act with Integrity

Reflection allows you to explore the integrity of your actions. In this reflection you would balance your values, principles, and codes against the outcomes to individuals, institutions, and communities. Acting with integrity preserves who you are throughout each situation. Usually seeking a middle ground option preserves your primary values. Even so there are some situations with no middle ground, killing an innocent human (murder), for instance. It could be suggested that removing extraordinary treatment so that an individual dies naturally from their illness is the middle ground between doing everything to try to save a person in a terminal condition and providing an intervention that kills.

Once you think you know what ought to be done, you need to check the impact of your actions. You need to consider the balance between positives in goods and benefits; and, the negatives in harms and costs. Sometimes one has to select the least harmful among harmful options, or the better or best among good options. As stated above, before you actually act on any ethical decision, you need to consider the impact of that action on all persons and institutions involved. It is essential that you consider imaginatively the impact of potential decisions on individuals and organizations impacted by the decision. This is looking at the potential good or harm to be done to each individual if you were to take your considered action. If you are acting as their surrogate, their advocate, put yourself in the place of the one for whom you are deciding. What would they want done? Put yourself in the place of your supervisor. How would they feel, what would they think about what you propose to do? What about your wife or husband or your parents, how would they feel, what would they think about this action? Would you want the story of your action placed in the newspaper? Finally, don't forget. To not act is still a chosen action. Many times, we are accountable just as much for what we do not do as for what we do.

You may have noticed that we have considered an integration of theories and models rather than promoting one position. This respects your individuality. The goal of this chapter and text is enriched decision-making capacity rather than the promotion of a position. It is our hope that you will gain insight into your valued principles and who you are so that you might act with integrity. The core of ethical decision making is listening carefully, thinking clearly and acting with integrity. Nonetheless, at this point your ethical development is still in process. We have made a good start, but there are areas not covered and ideas left to be discovered. It is hoped that you will continue to be reflective and build on these core ideas. You would be wise to stay open to new developments by considering yourself as learning and growing. The ideas and processes we have discussed will be enriched and strengthened as you think about them and relate them to your practice. In addition to this focus on your personal development, to be an ethically informed practitioner you need to be aware of common theoretical positions. This text has used Classical Virtue Ethics and Natural Law as organizing structures and sources of guiding principles. Additional ethical positions will be developed in the next chapter.

Sample Case with Ethical Analysis

What follows is a sample case developed for coursework. It is provided with analysis as a model for your consideration. This exercise will help clarify and develop critical thinking skills and hopefully continue to sharpen your ethical analysis:

The accountant-payroll clerk, Mr. J. D. is a single parent with two children at home. He has been a dependable, conscientious employee for ten years. During the last two months, though, he has missed six days of work for doctor's appointments and has made three serious errors on the payroll. There is concern that Mr. J.D.'s decline in productivity and increase in errors are affecting staff trust and the reputation of the whole department.

Mr. J.D. has lost weight, looks pale and has a cough. Other staff members have come asking if he has AIDS. As manager you have been answering, "I do not know." Last week in the performance interview, Mr. J.D. asked for some considerations because of his health. He confided that he has AIDS. He also asked that this be kept confidential. He says he has been having a temporary acute episode, is on medication and now feels much better. He is sure that his productivity and accuracy will return to its previous level.

Mr. J.D. needs to work to support his family. If known, he feels the information will jeopardize his ability to do his job and if he loses his position he will not have medical insurance. HIV/AIDS is a protected disability under the Americans with Disabilities Act[110], but Mr. J.D. is fearful there is still much discrimination.

Should the vice-president of finance be alerted? Should the manager cover for Mr. J.D. by asking other staff to do part of his work? Can the manager continue to say "I do not know" when asked? What alternatives would you suggest?

Listen to Your Self

Using the content just covered, you need to listen.

How do I feel about the request? Your self-talk may be the following:

"Wow, it would be hard for me. I wouldn't want to lose my job and insurance.

Being honest and open with employers has always been important to me.

Maybe this is just a temporary thing. If I agree to keep his confidence, I would have to do it. I keep my promises."

---

[110] https://www.ada.gov/ (accessed 02.15.19)

Listen to the Situation

In this situation, J.D. has a need to maintain employment, but his confidentiality request generates an ethical dilemma. Department staff are being asked to do extra work and suffer when other employees ask what has happened to their department. The department manager has to decide between concern for the human issues JD brings with his illness and his family, the law, concern for other employees, his loyalty to and responsibilities to his employer. The confidentiality request puts this manager in an awkward position.

Listen to Law, Codes, and Policies

There are policies about attendance. There are policies about work performance. It is against policy to cover up problems in a department. It is also against the law to discriminate against persons with AIDS. "The family and medical leave act"[111] may apply, but J.D. cannot afford to just take time off. We need to look into possible short- term disability programs, but there can be no accommodation without disclosure.

Listen to Principles

The principle of justice/fairness requires that I treat all employees the same. If I accommodate for J.D.'s absence and errors due to illness then I must accommodate C.A.'s tardiness due to child-care difficulties. Justice
also says that I must provide my employer with quality work. The principle of "Do unto other's what you would have them do unto you," says I need to make accommodation because that is what I would want.

Ask yourself, what is my ethical foundation? What are my values and virtue priorities? How do these fit within this situation?

Think Clearly

Experience and anticipating what Mr. J.D. was going to say helped the manager stay calm. Relevant ethical content includes concerns of how one ought to treat another person, i.e., confidentiality, truth-telling and being fair toward all. There is a desire to help the employee, to maintain confidentiality, to tell the truth, and to be fair to all employees and the division manager. They cannot all be done.

---

[111] https://www.dol.gov/whd/fmla/ (accessed 02.15.19)

Accommodation, short-term disability and the family leave act are available if J.D. is willing to share his needs with upper management.

In his youth the manager was taught to go the extra mile, to accommodate and help people. This conflicts with the need of a business to be run efficiently and with objectivity.

The manager is the primary decision-maker. He or she needs to establish priorities between these demands and develop a plan of action. Before acting, the manager needs to check the impact of possible decisions.

Check the Impact of Your Actions

Apparent Options

Covering for J.D. rather than Appraising VP of Situation

1. Impact on JD: Positive result; keeps his insurance, retains his job without fear.
2. Impact on staff: Negative result; asks other employees to do his share. May impact departmental morale. May lead other staff to expect leniency.
3. Impact on Division VP: Shown disrespect. Unable to plan, potential of surprise.
4. Impact on Manager himself: Violates his policy of honesty. Participating in deception.

Keeping Confidentiality rather than Breaking Confidentiality

1. Impact on JD: Unknown how VP will respond, JD would probably feel betrayed
2. Impact on staff: Allows for temporary staffing, if needed
3. Impact on VP: His right to information is fulfilled. Able to assist the department.
4. Impact on Manager himself: Retains his integrity, Avoids risk to his career from deception.

Middle Ground Options

From the previous analysis, it becomes clear that the VP must be informed or at least the manager cannot cover for JD. Since reaching this decision, two options become apparent to find the middle ground.

1. Provide JD with a short probationary period, say one month, after which if his work is not up to par the VP must be told JD is ill and the

department needs assistance. It is not essential that the nature of the illness be disclosed. Perhaps JD will make this contract.

2. Convince JD to go with you to the VP and discuss the situation with the VP. This will allow him to file for short-term disability and other benefits if they are needed and available. The advantage of short-term disability over the family act leave is continuing to receive pay.

Resolving an Ethical Dilemma

The ten questions that need to be answered in resolving an ethical dilemma: These assist with listening, thinking, sorting options, and acting with integrity.

1. Identify the ethical issues involved
2. What shows this is a moral dilemma?
3. What legal issue(s) are involved, this includes the law, codes and policies?
4. What is the apparent moral conflict? What principles are conflicting?
5. What are your conscience, cultural, and religious issues?
6. Who is responsible to make the decision and take action?
7. What are your personal conflicts and issues, especially if you are not the decision maker?
8. What additional knowledge is needed to make an informed decision? Consider the situation and persons involved, as well as the law.
9. What ethical principles, company policies, and codes impact what ought to be done?
10. Resolution: Provide a decision and its ethical rationale, which includes: a summary of the preceding content, options evaluated and their impacts, and the middle ground chosen.

Conclusion

Chapter Seven began with the need for virtue to move from the conclusion of what ought to be done to actually acting on the decision. The concluding decision is not enough. Typical responses to moral situations divide into six kinds of persons: the brute, the evil, the self-indulgent morally weak, the morally strong, the naturally moral, and the ideal individual. In order to do the good action, one must see he action as the good to be done in the situation. This insight requires a moral upbringing, knowledge of principles, the situation, and a decision of the good action. To move from the decision to actually make this good action requires virtue.

Virtue is a human excellence requiring knowledge and freedom. A moral action is a principle-based action towards the human good. For Plato, the Good is highest perfection and sustainer of the world that makes knowledge possible. Aristotle considered goodness a state of being that is excellent functioning for the kind of being under consideration. For humans this would be using reason and will to seek and choose the median behavior in the situation. Augustine held humans are in conformity with goodness when the right things are loved.

Ethical capacity grows as one reflects on situations, decisions, actions, and outcomes. Ethical dilemmas require one to move beyond reasoning of the practical syllogism and analogical reasoning comparing the current situation with landmark legal cases. An ethical dilemma can be resolved by attending to one's conscience, the situation, the law, codes, policies, and known ethical principles. Clear thinking is required to identify relevant content, values, principles and options in the situation. In acting, one will want to preserve personal and professional integrity. A sample case and its ethical analysis conclude the chapter.

Conversation Starters:

1. Individually or in a small group, make a list of examples where the moral has priority over the legal. Provide your rationale. Share examples with the class. Describe similarities and differences in examples discussed in class.

2. In your best judgment, what is required for a community to be at peace? Will this ever be achieved in the family? The health facility? Or, in society.

3. Thinking about the goodness being in the action or the outcome or both, where would you locate the goodness (if any) in the following:

Work on these with a partner then share your answers with the class.

   a. Assisting a blind person across a busy road.
   b. Pulling a struggling child out of a pool.
   c. Not stopping at a red light on a quiet street when late for work.
   d. Teaching third grade children long division.
   e. Maintaining confidentiality of an HIV+ test result for your friend's lover.
   f. Measuring radioisotopes carefully and providing the smallest radiation exposure.
   g. Completing the shift vital sign log, even though you did not have time to actually take all of the measurements.
   h. Sending a donation to the Red Cross.
   i. Working as a volunteer at the food pantry.

The good action for Aristotle is the median behavior, between extremes. What are the extremes and median for the above actions (1 a – i)?

Reflection Submissions:

1. Use Mr. JD and the framework provided as an example to resolve and write out a sample dilemma in your discipline, your life, or being in school. Use situations with issues other than confidentiality.

2. Use Aristotle's analysis of finding the median behavior with a moral question you have faced in your personal or professional life. Do you think this model of the median behavior leads to virtue? What virtue or virtues (include the four cardinal virtues, but there are others) are apparent in your example?

3. **Part one:** Augustine would consider the higher value to be the more immaterial option. What would Augustine say about the following:

   a. Having sufficient food and shelter or receiving free tuition

b. Having the freedom to attend the school of your choice or graduating from college without debt

c. Graduating from college without debt or being respected in the community

d. Receiving respect from family or from a health-care provider

e. Having good health or virtue

f. Doing satisfying work or controlling your own schedule

g. Being in a beautiful environment or listening to beautiful music

Part two: Rank the above Reflection options (1 a – g) based on your values. Explain your answers, supporting your choices.

Outline for Chapter 7: The Right Action Requires Discernment and Virtue

A. The Need for Virtue
    1. The four Cardinal Virtues
    2. Six characteristics human responses
    3. To see the good and do the good
    4. A virtuous action
    5. Finding the median
    6. A role model

B. Human Excellence
    1.The human good
        a. Augustine
        b. Aristotle

C. Ethical Decision Making
    1. Reflection grows ethical capacity
    2. Practical syllogism
    3. Analogical reasoning
    4. Ethical analysis

D. Confronting Ethical Dilemmas
    1. Listen carefully
    a. Listen to inner self
    b. Listen to situation
    c. Listen to the law, codes, and policies
    d. Listen to the sources of ethical principles
    2. Think Clearly
    a. Sorting options as a way of thinking
    3. Act with Integrity

E. Sample Case with Ethical Analysis
    1. Listen to yourself
    2. Listen to the situation

3. Listen to law, codes, and policies
4. Listen to principles
5. Think clearly
6. Check the impact of your actions
7. Apparent options
   a. Covering for J.D. rather than appraising VP of situation
   b. Keeping confidentiality rather than breaking confidentiality
8. Middle ground options
F. Resolving the Ethical Dilemmas
G. Conclusion

Terminology for Chapter 7
Moderation
Wisdom
Courage
Justice
Brute
Vicious
Weak-willed person
Strong-will person
Naturally moral person
Ideal person
Honorable
Beneficial
Legal
Consequentialism
Ethical dilemmas
Analogical reasoning

CHAPTER 8

A SHORT OVERVIEW OF PHILOSOPHICAL ETHICAL PERSPECTIVES

Objectives

This chapter provides an opportunity for you to:

1. Describe the human good and moral principles as provided in selected philosophical ethical perspectives.
2. Compare and contrast priorities of perspectives presented.
3. Identify perspectives complementary to your values and virtues.
4. Use presented perspectives in ethical analysis of moral situations.

Personal Moral Perspectives

This chapter will consider some philosophical ethical perspectives that enrich the caregiver's ethical analysis. The focus will include positions on the human good to be sought and the principles of action thought to bring the human good. First, we must consider personal moral perspectives. Resolving ethical questions begins with knowing yourself, your upbringing, and your tendencies to act or not act in different kinds of situations. Previous chapters have been concerned with these components of ethical inquiry. It was noted that values guide the acceptance or rejection of ethical principles. This is significant because principle-based actions are moral actions when they promote the human good. These chosen ethical actions will lead either toward goodness or at least away from a greater harm. Having integrity means the person you are is the person you take to school, home, and the workplace. The more unity there is between the person you are and what you are called to do in these settings, the more inner peace and personal satisfaction you will experience.

Moral Norms are One's Personal Standards of Behavior

Ethical norms are similar and closely related to moral norms, except, ethical norms are professionally based standards of action. They are often collected together as a profession's Code of Ethics. Ethical principles and moral norms can serve as a foundation for ethical decision making by providing the primary premise in the practical syllogism. While respecting moral norms and personal conscience, professionals need familiarity with selected philosophical ethical perspectives. Sources of moral norms include: parents and family; society and culture; religious/faith communities; elementary, secondary and college education; and, finally, what is modeled in music and on film. Most people just accept as moral what they have been taught or what they see people doing that "feels right" to them. When confronted with a situation, positive and negative feelings reflect what we have absorbed or grasped from our early childhood training. Feelings also reflect the habits we have developed. Positive or negative, right or wrong, good or evil, all previous actions mold what we feel ought to be done in the present. This feeling of right or wrong that is often called conscience and sometimes considered intuitive is strongly influenced by parents, friends, and culture. It could just be a parental voice, which means its trustworthiness depends on the moral quality of one's upbringing.

In youth and young adulthood, we become more alert to society, culture, and faith sources for how we ought to behave. We expand from a toddler wanting to please ourselves, to pleasing parents, to pleasing teachers, friends, even our pastor, priest, or God. Through our individual experiences, we develop a personal set of moral norms. Our moral choices arise from principles and ideas we value. These personal positions reflect our morality. Most people, either in their teens or early twenties, think they ought to decide right and wrong for themselves. They may or may not even accept legal limits on behavior.

Public Codes and Policies

Parents are usually happy when young people accept the law as behavioral norms. Nonetheless, moral norms or rules of behavior extend beyond the legal. As noted earlier in chapter six, the law is considered the minimum moral requirement. It is the least you can do to be a member of the community. Health practitioners add to obeying the law, "Do no harm" as their minimum moral standard. Ethics is the study of moral behavior considering what one should or ought to do (or not do). Ethics is also concerned with the study of morality and with public codes of behavior, the norms or rules for professions. These often translate into corporate policies or norms. Most corporate agencies have policy manuals. However, professional and personal codes may call the practitioner to follow a stricter standard than organizational policies. On the other hand, some organizational policies may be stricter than one's own code.

Virtue is achieved across time. Little by little good and peaceful choices lead to other good and peaceful choices. Who you are today is the culmination of who you have been. The choices you make today, small and large, generate who you will be tomorrow. Having a habit of doing the right action enables one to see the good to be done. Even so particular actions, right or wrong, may be a matter of some dispute. We have been structuring our work around humanity, so we have discussed the dignity of human life and how humans ought to be treated. We also noted the impact on the practitioner of professional care. Pellegrino teaches medical practice itself is a moral practice that increases moral awareness and virtue when the practitioner is striving to be an excellent physician.[112] Within our text, we have extended the concept of moral practice and its impact on the practitioner to include other health professionals. It is believed this statement would be agreeable to Pellegrino, since all health disciplines originate within the patient's need to maintain or recover their health through care-giver knowledge of patient need and applications of practice principles. This parallels the origin and goal of medical practice.

Philosophical Ethical Perspectives

Normative Ethics

Considered philosophically, acceptance of moral norms or rules outside of the personal desires of individuals leads to **normative ethics.** The ethical position that rejects external standards to argue the situation itself and the desires of the individual or culture determine the good to be done is called **relativism.** This is the first major division in the study of moral behavior (Ethics). Either one accepts that there are objective norms for human behavior or that there are not. Although many people like to argue that there are no standards, and that we are free to do whatever we want, they really only want that freedom for themselves. They do not want

---

[112] E. Pellegrino, "The Internal Morality of Clinical Medicine: A Paradigm for the Ethics of the Helping and Healing Professions," *Journal of Medicine and Philosophy,* 2001, (26:6) 559-579. (p. 560)

their neighbor to be allowed to take their things or throw stones at their house because the neighbor feels like it. Relativists often focus on tolerance asking for acceptance of those different from themselves in ideas and lifestyle. This focus on tolerance makes tolerance a norm or standard. Logic leads one to argue Relativism is self-contradictory because if one ought to be tolerant then there is a known standard by which one says, "We need to be tolerant of difference." In this way, relativism is a kind of normative ethics.

Professional codes help to specify ethical actions for the practitioner. They are imposed from the outside, from the perspective of the professional community. For example, physicians practicing within the **Hippocratic tradition** consider it their responsibility to tell the patient the best course of action. More contemporary physicians are likely to value patient **autonomy,** which is the patient's liberty to decide what is good for themselves. They explain options and encourage patients to participate in health-care decisions. Determining the proper human action from within the action itself recalls Pellegrino locating the physician's ethical call to action within the medical exchange (we would say, within the therapeutic relationship). This call to ethical action is found when patient vulnerability and the practitioner's educated capacity to intervene generate a responsibility for the practitioner.[113]

Emphasis on human excellence is the realm of virtue ethics, which was discussed extensively in Chapter Six. Determining the proper human action from what it means to be an excellent human being leads to valuing and promoting the virtues. The reader will recall the four cardinal virtues are wisdom, courage, moderation and justice. In Chapter Six we learned that virtue determines what is seen as a good action and that the median choice is usually the virtuous option. Aristotle referred to the median as the Golden Mean. We went through a process for finding the median. For situations when the practical syllogism and finding the mean are insufficient, we considered a set of steps for analysis of complex situations. These could be summarized as listening carefully, thinking clearly, and acting with integrity. Action grounded on what it is to be human in our complex world includes the perspectives of Thomas Aquinas' Natural Law Ethics and Immanuel Kant's Categorical Imperative. We considered Natural Law and the guidance it can provide in Chapter Seven. The shortest summary is that Natural Law Ethics[114] looks to what is eternal in human life, capacities of knowledge and freedom

---

[113] Ibid.
[114] Summa Theologicae, Q 93-97.

based on knowledge. Natural Law reasoning leads to the first principle of practical reason, to choose good and avoid evil. From this are derived three practical principles: (1) preserve human life, (2) educate the young, and (3) live in peace. These precepts are all required for one to seek truth and choose the good.

This chapter introduces the **Universal Moral Law** of Kant[115] and the contemporary perspective of T. L. Beauchamp and J. F. Childress[116] who propose four pillars of ethical action within professional practice called **Principlism**, the preservation of **beneficence**, **nonmaleficence**, **autonomy**, and **justice**. These four pillars or principles form an understandable structure for ethics, especially for students and practitioners new to ethical analysis, because they can be defined, accepted, and used in the practical syllogism. Nonetheless, it is possible they are not enough.

Additional theories included in this chapter are: **Utilitarianism,** J.S Mills[117] proposes evaluation and decision making based on agreeable consequences; and **Ethic of Care**[118] which finds moral guidance from within the web of relationships inherent in each ethical situation. While these are not a complete list of philosophical positions, they will provide the flavor and complexity of the study of right action and a range of positions within which you can further your ethical development.

Universal Moral Law

Kant is an eighteenth-century philosopher who seeks a moral standard by consideration of what it is to be human but came to very different conclusion from Aristotelian Virtue Ethics and from Aquinas' Natural Law. Kant realizes that humans are unique in reasoning capacity but that judgments influenced by experience are also influenced by personal preferences. He felt that to judge great moral leaders like Jesus Christ or Gandhi, one would have to have a higher standard as a basis of judgment.[119] He is seeking that standard. To escape bias, one would need to be reasoning outside of experience, reasoning from the meaning of the terms, i.e. being human, moral, and law. This absolute would be universal, meaning categorical, applying to all rational beings and the law would be

---

[115] *Grounding for the Metaphysics of Morals,* Trans. J.W. Ellington, Indianapolis, Indiana: Hackett Publishing Company, 1981.
[116] T. L. Beauchamp and J. F. Childress, *Principles of Biomedical Ethics.* New York: Oxford University Press, 2012.
[117] Stumpf, pp.372-379.
[118] www.iep.utm.edu/**care**-eth/ (accessed August 1, 2015)
[119] Kant, p.19-20.

followed from a morality of duty to the law itself rather than for another end. Hypothetical imperatives are for the sake of something else like, making a cake, having virtue, or being a member of a community. The foundation of the Moral Law is found in the unconditional value of being human. This value comes from our freedom and the ultimate value of a good will. Kant holds that a good will, one in conformity with the moral law, is the necessary condition of happiness, and of natural beings, humans are the only ones capable of this good will, good not in its outcomes but good in its willing to follow the moral law.[120] Because of his high estimate of what it is to be human, he taught that rational nature exists as an end in itself, Kant writes, "Everything in nature works in accordance with laws. Only a rational being has the power to act according to his conception of laws, i.e., according to principles, and thereby he has a will."[121] Kant asserts his moral imperative: "Act in such a way that you treat humanity, whether in your own person or in the person of another, always at the same time as an end and never simply as a means."[122] One has to ask, if you always treated humans as ends in themselves, how would you ever get checked out at the grocery store? We need each other for the services we provide. Clearly the answer is in the word 'merely.' Cashiers are a means for our completing our shopping and getting out of the store, but they are also being paid to perform this service. In a way, we are their means of feeding and sheltering. But Kant is very certain, "This principle of humanity and of every rational nature generally as an end in itself is the supreme limiting condition of every man's freedom of action."[123]

The Categorical Imperative of all rational beings is one ought to "act as if the maxim of your action were to become through your will a universal law of nature."[124] The principle of my action ought to be the principle of all free rational agents. Can I will that all persons act as I do (generalizability)? What impact would this have on society? Would I want to live in this community? Is this the way I would want to be treated (reversibility)? These questions are a restatement of the Golden Rule. The terms "generalizability" and "reversibility" have been added to highlight these important aspects of the Categorical Imperative. This same imperative is called Universal Law, Categorical Imperative or Moral Law. Even though there are different labels and phrasing, there is only one law.

Within the Kantian perspective, when faced with a tough ethical

---

[120] Ibid. p.7.
[121] Ibid. p.23.
[122] Ibid. p.36.
[123] Ibid. p.37.
[124] Ibid. p.30.

decision, you need to gain as much information as possible about the situation. Then consider an intervention, a principle of action that seems right to you based on your best judgment. With this principle in mind, one would look at the Universal Law and answer the above questions, repeated here: *Can I will that all persons act as I would with this principle of action? What impact would this have on society? Would I want to live in this community? Is this the way I would want to be treated*? If I could not will this generalized and reversible application, I cannot do the act. For some situations, it is clearer to see what ought to be done using the foundational application, am I treating others or my own person as an end or as a means to another end? Humans are the kind of being who ought to be treated as an end in themselves and never only as a means to an end.

Principlism

In the tradition of Plato, who required that lawmakers have knowledge of The Good in order to draft legislation with Justice, Beauchamp and Childress have promoted the view that in resolving moral dilemmas the practitioner needs to have knowledge of four principles and their applications.[125]

Nonmaleficence

The ancient medical maxim, "Above all, do no harm". This is the essential duty of anyone seeking to care for another. You can at least not harm them. The difficulty is that with some interventions there is always harm. Following a talk, I gave for physicians some years ago, a medical oncologist came up to me and asserted with some sorrow in his voice, everything I do causes some harm, but I cannot just let the patient die." Ronald Munson interprets Nonmaleficence to mean taking due care. He explains, "In effect, the principle of nonmaleficence tells us to avoid needless risk and, when risk is an inevitable aspect of an appropriate diagnostic test or treatment, to minimize the risk as much as is reasonably possible."[126]

Beneficence

This is the call to actively do something to intervene, to ameliorate the situation, to help the patient. Looking again to Munson, we read, "The duty required by the principle of beneficence is inherent in the role not only of physicians but of all health professionals. Nurses, therapists,

---

[125] See note 114.

[126] *Intervention and Reflection: Basic Issues in Medical Ethics, 5th ed.* Belmont, California: Wadsworth Publishing Company, 1995, p.34.

clinical psychologists, social workers, and others accept the duty of promoting the welfare of their patients or clients as an appropriate part of their responsibilities." It is the expectation that these professionals will do good for us that "leads us to designate them as belonging to what are often called 'the helping professions'."[127]

Autonomy

This principle follows the insight that humans are freely self-determined. This position is grounded in the human capacities of intellect and free will. Munson writes, "The principle of autonomy can be stated this way: *Rational individuals should be permitted to be self-determining.*"[128] Respect for autonomy (informed self-determination) is behind the requirements of informed consent. Health-care providers have responsibilities to inform patients about tests and interventions so they might make informed choices. Collaborative, mutual goal setting is a part of autonomy. Conditions that coerce patients, clients, or staff infringe on their autonomy signaling a moral violation.

Justice

In the health-care context, justice or fair treatment is generally concerned with distribution of goods and services. Again, reading from Munson for clarification, "Justice has at least two major aspects. Seeing to it that people receive that to which they are entitled, that their rights are recognized and protected, falls under the general heading of noncomparative justice. By contrast, comparative justice is concerned with the application of laws and rules and with distribution of burdens and benefits."[129] Non-distributive justice looks to the individual and to what they are entitled. Distributive justice is concerned with the whole community. This later involves access to health care and payment for services received. It is just that health-care providers receive compensation for services provided, but what happens when the patient has no money and no insurance? Justice is the moral principle governing allocation of scarce resources, even your time.

While acknowledging the need for accommodation, this system of ethical principles makes preservation of the principles themselves a goal. This leads to seeing them a bit 'other-worldly' in the Platonic sense. Nonetheless, the system is neat and accessible. When one has so many pressures, it is helpful to have a formula for right actions. Even though the system is limited, many well intentioned and moral practitioners depend on this model of ethical intervention.

---

[127] Ibid. p.34.
[128] Ibid. p.40.
[129] Ibid. p.37.

Utilitarianism

This is a very popular position today and it sounds wonderful. One only weighs the options and selects the option that brings happiness to the greatest number of persons. Your mother or father may have helped you make a difficult decision by having you list strengths and weaknesses of each option. This is very similar to seeking the most positive outcome for the whole community. Often one will total the number of persons who benefit or suffer less, but one may seek the outcome most beneficial to them. Neither of these were the intent of Bentham and Mills, his student. They sought a calculus to more easily determine the moral choice. Like many other scholars of the 18th Century, they were impressed by the power of mathematics. The goal was to make ethical decisions more mathematical so they would have greater certitude. The idea was a good one, except there are difficulties defining happiness. Bentham included all pleasures equally, while Mills called for human intellectual pleasures to be given a higher ranking. How do you compare eating with solving a great mystery?

Today students take "The persons who benefit from a decision" to be the individuals involved, but this was not the intent of the position. Bentham and Mills meant the benefit of the entire community. We are faced with questions as to whose benefit takes priority and what counts as a benefit or happiness? In a contemporary vein we ask, what brings the greatest happiness, a new housing complex or a ball field? How does one decide?

The contemporary utilitarian at Princeton, Peter Singer, would argue that the entire community includes all living things; that humans have no warrant to special treatment. He rejects the perspective that humans have a custodial responsibility for animals. In his view, we are all equal in pain, suffering and happiness. He takes reduction of the pain and suffering of the universe as the goal when resolving ethical conflict. With this in mind and with very gracious intent, he has famously recommended killing defective newborns because their lives would be filled with pain.[130]

Munson provides a positive utilitarian principle, *"We should act in such a way as to bring about the greatest benefit and the least harm."*[131] But, discussing this approach we just cannot escape questions of whose benefit, whose happiness.

---

[130] www.princeton.edu/~psinger/faq.html
[131] Munson, p.36.

Ethic of Care

Building on an analytic understanding of the human person provided by Aristotle and Aquinas, Clarke used phenomenology to emphasize human relationality. He taught that human fulfillment is found in transcendence of the self in communion with others. This perspective on human person is the relational message of an Ethic of Care. Most of the positions in this chapter have focused on human rationality, the human capacity to reason and reason's role in guiding ethical decision making, the ground of moral choice and human excellence. The last thirty years have seen a rise in the ethical acknowledgement of human relationships and the role of relationships in human development. Carol Gilligan's publication of her study on women facing crisis pregnancy, abortion, and child rearing revealed a very different moral development from the logic found in theories of justice.[132] Initially, it was believed that a woman's perspective with its emphasis on emotion, relationships, caring for others and interdependence rather than rationality, individuality and independence was totally different from the predominantly male model. Gilligan writes, "women perceive and construe social reality differently from men, and that these differences center around experiences of attachment and separation...because women's sense of integrity appears to be intertwined with an ethic of care, so that to see themselves as women is to see themselves in a relationship of connection, the major changes in women's lives would seem to involve changes in the understanding and activities of care."[133] This passage makes reference to understanding. As moral practice the Ethic of Care is not just intuitive or emotional, it requires knowledge and reasoning capacities. There needs to be a blend of wisdom and emotion, just as the rational capacities require the insight of emotion and the placement of the self within one's family and community relationships.

A full understanding of moral behavior requires insight into justice and human-rights based action and the role of emotion and relational interdependence. Knowledge of one's self and moral action requires the complementarity of these two perspectives. Annette Baier summarizes, "traditional justice-oriented ethics is inadequate. It masks inequalities among people, oversimplifies human relationships, and understates the moral importance of emotions like love. The best moral theory," she concludes, "must place care on an equal footing with justice."[134] Clearly

---

[132] *In a Different Voice.* Harvard University Press, 1982.
[133] *In a Different Voice*, p. 171 in J. Olen and V. Barry, *Applying Ethics: A text with Readings.* Belmont, California: Wadsworth Publishing Company, 1999. p. 43.
[134] 'The Need for More than Justice" in *Applying Ethics: a Text with Readings,*

Baier identifies some real difficulties with justice-oriented ethics. In contrast, concerns with a care-based ethics include the vulnerability of caring persons. Community-minded, tolerant, caring people are easily exploited. There is also reason for concern when some persons acting on emotion are willing to violate social norms. This tendency needs to be balanced with knowledge and self-restraint. The early emphasis on women and this being a feminist ethic has given way to the realization that both genders have emotional and rational aspects. Within this discussion personal integrity still includes a unity of being and doing. One needs to know themselves and act in ways consistent with who they are and who they want to be.

Conclusion

Students often say they do not want to evaluate what ought to be done because they do not want to think that they or a friend has done something wrong. They do not want to impose their beliefs on someone else. The irony is that you are more likely to do this unknowingly. The clearer you are on what your views are the easier it is to let the other person have their position. It is probably not possible to move through life without influencing others and imposing your beliefs in some way. Sometimes it seems the right thing to do is to stop so a driver can turn left in front of you into a driveway in the middle of the block; an expression of generosity. But when you stop you have imposed your values on the people behind you. Of course, if no one is behind you there is no reason to stop.

The following chart summarizes the ethical theories discussed:

Belmont California: Wadsworth Publishing Company, 1999. p. 41.

Position	Human good	Ethical principle (s)
Relativism	Personal freedom	Ever-changing moral world, but always have tolerance of others
Natural Law	Preserving truth and goodness	Do good, avoid evil Preserve human life Educate the young Live in peace
Categorical Imperative - Universal Law	Preserving good will Respecting humans	Act out of duty to CI/UL Chosen act must be generalizable and reversible All humans are ends in themselves
Virtue Ethics	An excellence of soul in conformity with reason	Preservation and development of the virtues
Principlism	Conformity with principles	Beneficence Nonmaleficence Autonomy Justice
Utilitarianism	Happiness	Evaluate consequences Greatest happiness/ good for the greatest number
Ethic of Care	Preserve relationships	Do what is needed to preserve relationships. Gives priority to those one cares about

Conversation Starters:
1. With all this emphasis on moral action and decisions towards the human good promoting peace and happiness, how do you explain why people suffer, even very moral virtuous people? Why is there not more peace and happiness?
2. It has often been argued that if you were starving or if you had starving children at home, it would be moral for you to steal food, or take a loan you know you will not be able to repay because life is the higher value. What would Kant say? Share your reasoning on his behalf using the Categorical Imperative and the foundation in how rational beings ought to be treated. Consider especially what taking the food or money says about the grocer or banker from whom the items are taken.
3. As a patient, would you choose to be taken care of by someone who focused on justice and rights-based care or someone who focused on relational caring-based care?
4. Parenting stresses relationships between unequal persons. Identify and evaluate rights-based and care-based requirements of parenting.

Reflection Submissions:
1. Place yourself as confronted with an ethical situation to which you must respond. Write out the situation. Compare suggested actions using (1) Virtue Ethics, (2) Natural Law Ethics and (3) Kant's Categorical Imperative with (4) its foundation on how one ought to treat all rational beings.
2. Consider suggested actions for the above ethical situation from a Utilitarian perspective, Relativism, and an Ethic of Care.
3. This is a good time to compare and contrast your discipline's code of ethics with your personal list of moral norms.
4. Explain why you would choose to be taken care of by someone who focused on justice and rights-based care or someone who focused on relational caring-based care.

Outline for Chapter 8: A Short Overview of Philosophical Ethical Perspectives
A. Personal Moral Perspectives
    1. Moral norms are one's personal standards of behavior
    2. Public codes and policies
B. Philosophical Ethical Perspectives
    1. Normative ethics

Terminology for Chapter 8
Morality
Normative
Relativism
Hippocratic tradition
Universal Moral Law
Principlism
Beneficence
Nonmaleficence
Autonomy
Justice
Utilitarianism
Ethic of Care
Hypothetical Imperative
Categorical Imperative

SECTION FIVE:

HUMANITY AT THE HEART OF PRACTICE

It is the position of this book that your view of human life stands behind what is seen as an issue in personal and professional ethics, what generates an ethical dilemma, and what resolves it. For this reason, after considering values, their impact in our lives, and good argumentation, we began with a classical perspective of human life as substantial and relational. Personal and professional ethical behaviors are human actions based on principles, either as conscious decisions or from habit. We have been asserting that as virtuous persons, these principles need to be in our awareness and shown to promote the human good. Professionals need to also follow expectations of their disciplinary codes, as well as the law and corporate policies. Ethical practice takes into account the individuality of each person and calls professionals to be aware of cultural and religious values. These values are an integral part of human transcendence, governing our sense of morality.

In Section Four, we considered decision making and foundational principles from philosophical inquiry that can become the primary premise in a practical syllogism that resolves the dilemma and moves the health-care professional toward action. While studying Section Five, you are invited to review your work in earlier chapters. A significant goal might be by the completion of this section you will have a set of studied positions and rationales that make a coherent whole of moral action and professional practice. Every effort has been made to present views from both sides of debated issues like abortion and euthanasia. Where scientific information is available and adds to our understanding for ethical-decision making, it is provided. It is desirable that you thoughtfully engage in discussion of these topics critical for the informed practitioner.

If we assert ethical behavior respects human life, we still need to know what human life is, when it begins, and when it ends. And we need to know the characteristics of an action that is respectful of life. It is not possible to anticipate all ethical decisions with which you will be confronted. This section will provide opportunities to further develop your knowledge of issues and your reasoning capacities for analysis and decision making. With these positions, rationales, and capacities you will have tools for resolving future ethical dilemmas.

Chapters Nine and Ten directly address human life in its origins and as it ends. Beginning of life issues require that we make the distinction between the living and non-living, the human and the non-human. End of life and palliative care make the additional distinction between killing and letting die. At both the beginning and end of life, discussions ask if full moral rights are attached to all humans or just those meeting certain criteria like self-consciousness. Chapter Eleven considers the professional within practice issues interfacing with other professionals, patients, and health care institutions within the larger community.

CHAPTER 9

ETHICAL ISSUES RELATED TO THE BEGINNING OF LIFE

Objectives

This chapter provides an opportunity for you to:

1. Explore moral and legal accountability with different levels of involvement in issues at the beginning of life.
2. Describe options for when human life begins.
3. Explore scientific and philosophical reasons for and against select positions on issues at the beginning of life, like abortion, IVF, cloning, and embryonic stem cell research.
4. Evaluate your proposed positions on issues at the beginning of life.

Moral and Legal Accountability

A Personal Experience

In the mid-1970s, while working clinically as temporary staff, I had the following experience. The patients on my assigned unit were all women. It was designated GYN (gynecology). I had worked some on the OB floor (obstetrics) but not so often on GYN. Most of the patients had a hysterectomy or D & C, but one of my patients, a young woman of sixteen, was preparing for surgery in the early afternoon. I was told she was having a saline procedure. I had "no clue." A fellow nurse explained, "The surgeon would remove amniotic fluid and replace it with a strong saline." I asked, "What will that do to the baby?"

"Kill it," she said, bluntly. She continued, "A few hours after her return from the operating room, she will go into labor and deliver a dead baby, which is what she wants."

"Is that legal?" I asked.

"Yes, it's legal; abortion is legal in all states since 1973," she continued. "This is a late, second trimester abortion, and this doctor will do saline abortions quite late; 6 ½ or 7 months." How naïve I was! I had been a nurse for ten years and somehow, I had missed that abortion kills a baby. I understood that abortion ends a pregnancy, but I did not make the connection. I just didn't think about it. I was told to obtain the consent but to not say much about the procedure; just that the doctor will instill saline solution.

In 1970, I had driven a friend from Massachusetts to New York. What she needed was legal in New York City. At the time, I did not realize we were going to an abortion clinic. I just knew she needed a ride, and I had a car. In the car she told me she had made a mistake and needed to fix it. She told me she'd be an hour or so. I need not come in. She suggested I just get some toast while waiting because lunch would be too expensive. She was right! We focused on the expense of New York City and ignored what was happening. She seemed "shaken" when she returned. I asked if she was okay and accepted her answer. "I'm okay; let's just get home so I can lie down in my own bed." We didn't talk much. When home she said, "I'm glad that's over, I won't let that happen again."

Silly me, I say. "Don't worry; I was glad to give you a ride." I must have been "sleepwalking." I was really not in touch with what was happening.

This New York event came clearly to my mind at the women's unit speaking with this frightened young lady having the saline abortion. As expected, she went into labor and delivered a stillborn baby. She was filled with distress, "I can't believe it. I had the abortion because I was afraid of labor and they made me go through labor" … and on and on. It was really sad. She said, "If I'd known I had to go through labor, I would have had the baby." The little one was quite large. He almost did not fit into the jar in the nurse's station. I was deeply grieved and quit my job the next day. Before leaving, I asked a nurse who had worked there for a long time why she stayed. How did she deal with this? She told me she was Catholic and did not believe in abortion but stayed to baptize the babies. She said sometimes they were born alive, and she got to take them to the newborn nursery. Another person told me she only worked in the nursery and ignored this aspect of the hospital.

An Experience of Socrates

The *Crito* is a short dialogue written by Plato on behalf of his mentor, Socrates, who had been convicted and sentenced to death for corrupting the youth and not believing in the city's gods. This discussion between

Socrates and his friend Crito explains Socrates cannot escape into exile to save his life. By remaining in Athens for his whole life, Socrates had an implied agreement to obey the laws of the city. Even though Socrates was falsely accused and unjustly convicted, by escaping into exile Socrates would violate his contract with the city undermining its laws. In this, he would be supporting his conviction. He would be corrupting the youth, who following Socrates' example, may not respect the laws throwing the city into chaos. The underlying principle of Socrates' action was, it's never right to do wrong, even if one has been wronged.[135] Today one often hears, "Two wrongs do not make a right." While an important maxim, our focus is implied consent.

Implied Consent

Hospitals do much to enrich human life and to bring health and comfort to people. It could be said quitting my job was over-reactive. One has to consider if staff not directly participating in a procedure are morally responsible. Are laboratory, x-ray, and health records personnel accountable for patient care in a hospital? Are they consenting to procedures done within the hospital?

Guilt by association has gotten many people into difficulty. For example, a young woman was grateful to land a well-paying job in dentistry. She had been a dental assistant for years, but in this position she was in-putting data for patient accounts. She was offered a handsome salary. She began to notice that many patients had credit on their accounts and charges for work that was not done. This bothered her a bit, but the dentist explained that billing this way kept the patients from having to pay large bills, and anyway, they might need the work in the future. The young woman decided that she would have to give up this great job, with its great salary, because staying would imply she agreed with the dentist's illegal practices.

A few months later the dentist was in prison for insurance fraud. If she had retained the job she would have gone to court and might have been convicted as an accessory. Individual accountability would not allow her to plead that she was just following the dentist's instructions. She was the one in-putting the data. She had a responsibility to know what she was doing. Other members of the office were investigated, but only the new

---

[135] 49a-d, in *The Trial and Death of Socrate*, 3rd edition. Translated by G. M. A. Grube and revised by J. M. Cooper, Indianapolis: Hackett Publishing, 2000. pp. 43-54.

data secretary was tried with the dentist. The person was not convicted as there was cause to believe she did not fully grasp what she was doing since she had just begun the position.

One has to ask, how closely involved do you have to be to be morally accountable? Does paying taxes make one responsible for what Congress decides on behalf of the country? Does letting a friend borrow your gun reflect on you when it is used to rob the bank? Does it make a difference whether or not the intent to rob the bank was known? Does driving to New York City for your friend to obtain an abortion make you partially responsible for the death of the fetus? Does it make a difference whether or not the driver knew her friend's intent? There are many facets to these experiences. In-vitro fertilization (IVF), embryonic stem cell research, and cloning all raise abortion questions because of discarding or killing embryos. When is it acceptable to sacrifice one human for another? In the **self-defense argument,** when one person endangers another, the innocent may morally protect his or her life even if the other is killed. It seems, this argument can justify the loss of the fetus. Another way of reasoning is from the **principle of double effect**, which holds that a person may morally perform an action that he foresees will produce a good effect and a bad effect provided that four conditions are verified at one and the same time:

1. that the action in itself from its very object is good or at least indifferent;
2. that the good effect and not the evil effect is intended;
3. that the good effect is not produced by means of the evil effect;
4. that there is a proportionately grave reason for permitting the evil effect.[136]

At the beginning of life, a fetus may morally be removed from a fallopian tube because leaving it there will result in rupture as the fetus becomes larger than space available. The mother will die from the resulting hemorrhage, and the fetus will also die. The goal is not death of the fetus but preserving the life of the mother, which is the intended good end. Either way the fetus dies.

With abortion procedures the intent is to kill the unborn human. The underlying questions are when does human life begin? What dignity or respect is owed a molecular embryo? And when does the new being

---

[136] Mangan, Joseph (1949). "An Historical Analysis of the Principle of Double Effect," *Theological Studies*, 10: 41–61. From
http://plato.stanford.edu/entries/double-effect/ (accessed August 18, 2013.)

acquire full moral standing with human rights and the inherent right to life?

Acquiring Protection of Human Rights

The human rights asserted in the preamble (2.1) of the United States Declaration of Independence reads, "We hold these truths to be self-evident, that all men are created equal, that they are endowed by their Creator with certain inalienable rights, that among these are life, liberty and the pursuit of happiness."[137] These are expanded to humanity as a whole through the United Nations Declaration of Human Rights. From today's perspective, it seems human rights are well established in the United States. But it has been just over fifty years since racial minorities and women won legally protected equal opportunity in education and the workplace.[138] It was during the 1960's Civil Rights Movement that laws establishing Child Protective Services were passed by Congress to prevent abuse, exploitation, and neglect.[139] Two hundred years of development were required to extend the natural law expressed in the Declaration of Independence to provide full moral standing for men, women, and children.

Human rights, theoretically extended to all humans, raise the difficulty whether or not a particular individual is a bearer of rights. Foundational to all of these rights is the right to life because one must be alive to do anything else; either being free or seeking happiness. Within this chapter, we ask if asserting all humans deserve the right to life includes the unborn at every stage of development. In the next chapter, we ask the same question about those in a coma.

When Human Life Begins

Chapters Three and Four provided information on human life, including its beginning, within the contemporary Aristotelian-Thomistic tradition which updates classical philosophy with contemporary science. We considered substantial beings in nature as matter/form unities. For living beings, the form is the nature of the thing or person. The presence of

---

[137] http://users.wfu.edu/zulick/340/Declaration.html (accessed August 9, 2013)
[138] http://www.infoplease.com/spot/womenstimeline1.html and
http://www.infoplease.com/spot/bhmtimeline.html (accessed August 17, 2013)
[139] http://www.americanbar.org/content/dam/aba/publishing/insights_law_society/
ChildProtectionHistory.authcheckdam.pdf (last accessed December 30, 2018)

the actualizing form signals the presence of the being of a particular kind. For humans the internal principle of activity and rest is clearly present at human genome activation at approximately 52 hours after the sperm reaches the ovum. In the four-cell stage of the zygote one cell "switches on." This spark that initiates self-development is called human genome activation.[140] From this moment the new DNA, formed by intertwining of the maternal and paternal chromosomes, assumes functions of development starting with generation of its own messenger RNA. We do not use "all development" because environmental factors impact which potentialities within the chromosomes are available to the new individual. This complex mechanism of chromosome selection is not fully understood, nonetheless, the spontaneous shift in the zygote to its own principle of activity and rest signals a time beyond which one cannot deny the generation of a new human being. Aristotle calls this generation of a new being substantial change. The parents are human, and the new being is human with its own intellectual soul and the potential for self-consciousness.

Because of the contemporary emphasis on personhood, we are left to ask, "Is the beginning of a new human life the same as the beginning of a new personal life? Is the multicellular living being with human DNA, which is the human molecular embryo, a bearer of human rights? Do these molecular humans have moral standing?" It is very clear within the contemporary science of Human Molecular Embryology that the zygote making human DNA is alive and is human, but the question remains, "Is being alive sufficient to warrant the respect of human rights?"

Many individuals assert extra-mental reality (the world outside of the mind) to be the way they *want* it to be rather than the way *it is*. Confronted with difficult implications, we often prefer to stay with the way we believe the world is (belief) rather than knowledge, even if alternative facts disputing our beliefs are available. And, we seem to want to allow people the 'reality' they prefer, so they can do what they want unopposed. On the contrary, as difficult as it is, we assert truth (what actually is the case) provides real freedom, because you need to know truth to have real

---

[140] Whelton, "On the Beginning of Human Life," *Linacre Quarterly,* February 1998, 51-65, "Human Nature, Substantial Change, and Modern Science: Rethinking When a New Human Life Begins," lecture, The American Catholic Philosophical Association, March 28, 1998. Published in the Proceedings, Vol. LXXII, 1999, pp. 305-313. Further discussion may be found in the work of Robert P. George and Patrick Lee, Embryonic human persons. Talking Point on morality and human embryo research. EMBO Reports 2009 Apr; 10(4): 301–306. https://www.ncbi.nlm.nih.gov/pmc/articles/PMC2672893/

choices. Arguments for abortion, in vitro fertilization (IVF), cloning, and stem cell research often center around the human ability to provide the procedure and the apparent right to do what suits us. The attitude is, "If we can do it, it must be moral; God would not allow a procedure that was wrong." There is a strong desire to do what we want especially that which provides solutions to problems, including social problems. In the next section of this chapter, we will further define life and personhood to consider what these definitions contribute to this discussion.

Defining Life

Contemporary Aristotelian understandings see no division between the natural form of the body and the human rational soul. Rationality is the highest capacity of the human intellectual form. Within Aristotle's text, *On the Soul*[136], he taught the human form was the rational soul. This contrasts to his delay in ensoulment[141] where males are asserted to be living at 40 days after the sperm enters the ovum and females at 90 days. The writings of Aquinas, Aristotle's medieval commentator, refer to quickening, when movement is first detected, as showing life. In the *Politics,* Aristotle wrote that the state ought not to allow abortion after motion can be detected because this motion indicates a new living human.[142] Contemporary science shows there is self-movement in the molecular embryo, calling us to acknowledge along with human molecular embryologists, that the new human is alive. Nonetheless, these embryologists do not accept this molecular embryo as a human being, just human tissue.

In contrast to early **hominization** with matter/ form unity, there are consequentialist reasons for holding a dualist view of the soul. If we are physical beings, which at some point receive an indwelling soul, then we can have a living human biological being which does not have an intellectual soul and thus is not yet human. This allows for procedures prior to ensoulment, and after the loss of self-consciousness, that one would not accept being done to a human person. In this perspective, the molecular embryo and fetus at certain stages of development can be said to be human but do not have human rights. Human rights become reserved for those identified as persons.

---

[141] http://abortionmedicalethics.weebly.com/when-is-a-fetus-considered-alive.html (accessed January 17, 2015).
[142] *Politics,* in McKeon, pp. 1302.

Personhood

In the development of the embryo and fetus, there are capacities expressed that seem to move the individual close to personhood, but when is it a person? If an embryo is not a person from the beginning of its existence as a living being, one has to ask when the embryo becomes a person.

As referred to earlier in chapter four, the sixth century philosopher Boethius provides the classic definition of person as "an individual substance of a rational nature."[143] Philosophers hold different times for the fulfillment of Boethius' definition: (1) some accept conception because of the origination of a new living being; (2) some accept **individuation,** the time beyond which the embryo can no longer be twins, approximately seven days; (3) in consideration of **rationality**, some hold the development of primal streak, the earliest cell differentiation anticipating neurons at twelve days; (4) others consider the necessary factor to be the beginning of heart beats at 4 weeks; (5) and others establishment of the brain at twelve weeks. The difficulty in accepting any of these events is that there is no apparent change in kind from genome activation to death. There is growth and development with expression of capacities, but these can be seen as included potentials within the DNA of the zygote.[144] There is good reason to hold with the second century philosopher, Tertullian (160-220 AD), that what will be human is human.[145] Not all human zygotes will mature into infants, but they do not become something else. All infants were formerly human zygotes. Humans only come from humans. If one accepts Tertullian's view, then all humans have human rights. The new individual comes into existence with the right to life.

Gregory E. Pence[146] disagrees that human moral rights and human life both begin with activation of the molecular embryonic genome. He separates acceptance as human life from acceptance as having full moral standing and provides an analysis of the moral status of the unborn from the 1973 Supreme Court Decision, Roe v. Wade. Pence's passage reads as follows:

> The court decided that the moral value of a human mother is that of a full person, but that of an 8-day human embryo is minimal. As the embryo grows to become a fetus, its moral value grows. At birth, its moral value or standing matches that of its mother.

---

[143] http://www.newadvent.org/cathen/11726ahtm (assessed August 10, 2013).
[144] See note 138.
[145] http://www.religioustolerance.org/abo_when4.htm (accessed January 17, 2015).
[146] Pence, *The Elements of Bioethics,* Boston, McGraw Hill, 2007. p. 176.

This analysis implies, as the Court ruled, that during the first two trimesters (weeks 1-13 and 14-26), the Mother's interest outweigh that of the fetus and that abortions can be justified. Of great importance to ethical reasoning, the analysis implies that as the moral value of the fetus increases, the reasons needed to justify aborting it become more demanding. This is why using a morning-after pill to prevent a 2-day old embryo from implanting in the uterus requires much less justification than a very late-term abortion of a fetus at 37 weeks.[147]

Pence's analysis shifted the emphasis from being human to being a person having moral standing. The Declaration of Independence uses the language of being human, even though at the time it meant only land-owning males. As we read it today, there is nothing that says person. We question how this shift from human to person happened. Pence used the criteria of Mary Anne Warren, "to be a person is to be able to think, to be capable of cognition."[148] She feels all first and second trimester abortions are justifiable because the fetus does not meet this criterion of being able to think, so while a human is lost, no person is killed.

In 2004, the President's Council on Bioethics debated potentiality and personhood in discussing medical research on human embryos. The Council's chair, Leon Kass, argued that these embryos' potential for personhood conferred moral value on them. A dissenting member of the Council, Dartmouth neuroscientist Michael Gazzaniga, made the analogy that, "Even though a Home Depot may contain the supplies to build a dozen homes, when a Home Depot burns down, we do not say that a dozen homes were destroyed."[149] In other words, a potential person is not a person.

Symmetry between the Beginning of Life and the Declaration of Death

Writing in his text, *The Basics of Bioethics,* Robert M. Veatch proposes there is symmetry between the three common definitions of death with loss of moral standing and determination of the beginning of full human moral standing with its right to life.[150] Perhaps Veatch's considerations will shed some light on our effort. One's position on the definition of death could determine one's position on defining human life.

---

[147] Ibid.

[148] "On the Moral and Legal Status of the Fetus," *The* Monist 57 (1973), pp. 43-61.in Pence, p. 178.

[149] Carl Zimmer, "Michael Gazzaniga: Scientist at Work," *The New York Times,* May 12, 2005, p. D3 in Pence, p.178).

[150] Third edition, Boston: Pearson Education Inc., 2012. Chapter Three, "Defining Death, Abortion, Stem Cells, and Animal Welfare: The Basis of Moral Standing," pp. 25-46.

Cardiac Declaration of Death

The historical Cardiac-oriented declaration of death with its irreversible loss of cardiac and respiratory function would lead one to accept that the embryo has full moral standing when capacity for cardiac function appears. There then emerges the question of the meaning of cardiac function, beating or pumping. As noted earlier, heart beats begin at approximately four weeks, but pumping much later at eight weeks.[151]

Whole-brain Criteria of Death

The Harvard criterion of whole brain death, with its irreversible loss of all functions of the entire brain, implies full moral standing occurs with appearance of neurological integration at eight to twelve weeks.

Higher Brain Death as a Criterion

A contemporary view under debate, higher brain death is irreversible loss of consciousness, which withdraws full moral standing from patients with persistent vegetative state, end-stage dementia, and traumatic injury with minimal brain function. This position takes the body to be living to some degree as supported by health care, but the person is gone. Pence considers this individual a person-absent body.[152] In this view health care providers are doing harm by maintaining a dead body. Veatch suggests holders of this view would attribute full moral standing to a fetus with the appearance of higher brain function at approximately twenty-four weeks.

Higher brain function is said to be consciousness of self and other bodily functions. This seems hardly possible at twenty-four weeks, and usually cannot be said of the newborn. This position of higher brain function supports the recent famed proposal of after-birth abortion.[153] The two professors writing in the *Journal of Medical Ethics*, Alberto Giubilini and Francesca Minerva, propose that since neither fetuses nor newborns have capacities that warrant full moral standing and are only potential persons, there is no reason to prohibit killing the newborn if it is a burden on the family. This has nothing to do with a defective newborn, just a sense of burden, financial or social, similar to how one may argue about a

---

[151] https://www.whattoexpect.com/pregnancy/fetal-development/fetal-heart-heartbeat-circulatory-system/
[152] Pence, p.140.
[153] http://jme.bmj.com/content/early/2012/03/01/medethics-2011-100411.full (accessed August 10, 2013).

woman's need for and right to access abortion. In effectively applying the strongest pro-choice arguments to killing the newborn, they got world-wide attention and called other academics to question what is being said of fetuses.

Veatch and Pence are attributing moral standing based on certain capacities, rather than on being human. Who makes these decisions? Is moral standing a stable norm? We have seen progression in legal protections of natural rights grounded on the Declaration of Independence. The critical question is whether humans have moral rights, or if you have to be human plus additional attributes, like being self-conscious, to have these moral rights. The Supreme Court in Roe v Wade said one must have certain attributes. One has certain minimal rights at conception with full moral rights at birth. It is important to notice the switch from humans having rights to humans of certain capacities having rights. This discussion asks us to take seriously our position on the body-soul relationship, what generates personhood, and the moral acquisition of the right to life.

The haunting question remains, "Who's in charge of life?" We wonder if there is a design and a designer. Is life the product of evolution and thus, chance? Perhaps there was a designer, but he or she left control of human life up to humans. How to decide? If there is a designer, how can we best cooperate with the plan, the design, to the extent it can be known. This effort builds on Natural Law Ethics, which we discussed in Chapter Seven.

The scholar, James A. Donald wrote an excellent account of Natural Law and Natural Rights justified within an evolutionary context. He argues that "the ability to make moral judgments, the capacity to know good and evil, has immediate evolutionary benefits: just as the capacity to perceive three dimensionally tells me when I am standing on the edge of a cliff, so the capacity to know good and evil tells me if my companions are liable to cut my throat."[154] Consistent with the position that all good persons can make moral judgments, Donald does not require a designer.

The Informed Decision

The intent of this chapter is to provide enough information for you to make an informed decision on whether or not you would have an abortion or support your friend in procuring an abortion. This has been a complex topic to explore. There are definite areas of knowledge required to make an informed decision; like when the new being has a soul and when an

---

[154] http://jim.com/rights.html (Accessed August, 16, 2013).

individual acquires full moral rights. Philosophically, it is not desirable that you just accept a position because someone else does. The good can be known by both secular and religious experts, though their views do not, in themselves, make a position or action moral. Perhaps the most important requirement of a moral action is whether or not it promotes the human good. Is the human good upheld by sacrificing a vulnerable class of humans for another class of humans? Is the human good supported when an upwardly-mobile, gifted woman sacrifices herself for a tiny defective human or even a seemingly perfect one? It may be that a mother's love for her child changes the degree the unborn is valued. But it does not change who the fetus is and its human rights. Surely, something about the perspective changes the little one from being a difficulty to being cherished by the mother, but not its being human. That does not change.

Impact of Technology

The three topics to now be addressed are the gift and curse of modern science. Considering their potential to improve fertility and aspects of human health, one would say gift, but challenges to the dignity of human life lead some to consider them a curse. Just like human dissection within the Renaissance, these scientific advances challenge the intersection of faith and science. Philosophically, one must be willing to consider difficult topics and to be open to reasonable arguments. Even if one decides to reject the conclusion as violating their faith, one can acknowledge the strengths and weaknesses of contrasting positions. Part of being an educated person is learning to treat those who agree or disagree with our positions with respect. In discussion, you are expected to provide reasoned arguments with premises in support of your conclusions. These topics grounded in technology offer opportunities for thoughtful discussion in which we evaluate arguments and not the person expressing the argument.

In-vitro fertilization (IVF)

In-vitro means in the lab, in the test tube. It contrasts with in-vivo, in a living organism, in the natural setting. IVF is a technologically assisted method of generating an embryo. This embryo may be for agricultural use to raise animals with desired traits, like high milk production, or for solving difficulties with human infertility. Bradley J. Van Voorhis reports that, "in 2003, more than 100,000 IVF cycles (ova stimulation, harvesting, fertilization, embryo growth and implantation) were reported from 399 clinics in the United States, resulting in the birth of more than 48,000 babies (parenthetical content added)."[155] Within the natural course of human reproduction there is a 20% chance that a fertilized ovum will reach implantation. Once implanted, there is an 80% chance the pregnancy will come to live birth. With IVF fresh non-donor eggs, the average pregnancy rate in 2003 was 34% implantation, with 28% resulting in live birth.[156]

IVF can overcome the effects of age with the use of donor eggs. A woman 34 years old using IVF procedure to become pregnant with her own ova will have 40% to 49% chance of a live birth. However, at age 43 with IVF and her own ova, the woman has a 5% chance of live birth from each pregnancy. The percent of live births per pregnancy returns to near 50% with donor ova from a young woman. Clearly, IVF represents an effective way for an older woman to achieve pregnancy but markedly diminished live births unless donor eggs are used.

Moral Considerations of IVF include Financial and Human Costs

The cost for each cycle is $10,000 to $20,000 with most pregnancies requiring more than one cycle. Because of the cost and simply the stress and risk of procedures, multiple embryos may be placed in the uterus for implantation. In this way IVF can result in multiples; twins, triplets, and more. Parents also have the option to have any remaining embryos frozen for future use.

Kant (1724-1804) holds humans have dignity, inner worth, because of our human potential to develop a good will, which is the minimal requirement for happiness. When Kant says, in his moral philosophy that an individual has, "either a price or a dignity,"[157] the impression is given we ought not to buy and sell humans. Yet, while it is true that IVF costs parents large sums of money, so does an adoption procedure.

Implantation of multiple embryos leads to pregnancy reduction (abortion of some fetuses) or multiple births with very low weight premature births (less than 1500 grams, a bit more than 3 pounds). The premature births scenario results in high potential for pulmonary and neurological dysfunction. Even with a single implantation, IVF children

---

[155] "In Vitro Fertilization", www.nejm.org New England Journal of Medicine 356:4, January 25, 2007, p. 379. (accessed August 10, 2013).

[156] This is written with an awareness that scientists have continued research to increase quality of the embryo implanted to enhance the number of live births. We have stayed with older, simpler data to show the contrast between non-IVF and IVF and impact of age.

https://www.sartcorsonline.com/rptCSR_PublicMultyear.aspx?ClinicPKID=0

[157] *Groundwork of the Metaphysics of Morals,* translated and edited by Mary Gregor. NY: Cambridge, 1998, pp. 42-43.

have lower birth weight and an increased tendency towards birth defects.

For Aristotle, rationality is the highest known capacity in our world, and gives human's value. We have asked before, "Can rationality be a natural capacity? Could it be that an immaterial capacity like reasoning with immaterial concepts and self-reflection requires an immaterial source?" This immaterial source cannot be found in nature. If it is true that the unique human capacities of intellect and will are given supernaturally to each person at conception, it is possible humans ought to respect God's plan for human generation. Even so, a child conceived through technology is still a human child and worthy of respect and human rights. We argue that regardless of one's beginnings, natural or artificial, if a live embryo results, God provided an intellectual soul.

The apparent ethical concerns of IVF are: abortion of unwanted embryos, cryopreserving or discarding of extra embryos, the impact of apparent buying and selling human life, and the just use of finances. For some, the issue of human interference in conception is significant. Intimacy between men and women is directed toward new life as its natural fulfillment.

Cloning

Cloning is asexual reproduction. This occurs in nature with some plants and animals.

Researchers make copies of genes they want to study. They will place genetic material they want to study into unicellular organism, like a yeast or bacterium. They then use minute electrical or chemical stimulation to encourage the intended new combination to begin cell division and growth. This is the process by which scientist provided Humulin insulin from e. coli bacteria. This insulin carries greater efficiency and fewer negative side effects than the use of insulin from beef or pig pancreatic Islet cells.

The National Human Genome Research Institute of the National Institutes of Health (NIH) makes available a cloning fact sheet. We read, "In reproductive cloning, researchers remove a mature somatic cell, such as a skin cell or an udder cell, from an animal that they wish to copy. They then transfer the DNA of the donor animal's somatic cell into an egg cell, or oocyte, that has had its own DNA-containing nucleus removed."[158] This can be done through nuclear transfer or by fusing the two cells together.

---

[158] "Cloning" http://www.genome.gov/25020028 (last accessed December 31, 2018).

The egg is allowed to develop into an early embryo and is implanted into the uterus of the host animal. Mammals that have been cloned include: cat, deer, dog, horse, mule, ox, rabbit and rat. Agricultural animals may also be reproduced through the simple process of twinning, splitting an embryo.

You may be familiar with Dolly, the cloned lamb. We read, "It was not until 1996, however, that researchers succeeded in cloning the first mammal from a mature (somatic) cell taken from an adult animal. After 276 attempts, Scottish researchers finally produced Dolly, the lamb, from the udder cell of a 6-year-old sheep. Two years later, researchers in Japan cloned eight calves from a single cow, but only four survived."[159] The NIH report[160] goes on to describe serious drawbacks, one being the 276 failed attempts, others include the increased birth size and defects in vital organs, like heart, liver, and brain. It is also of some importance that Dolly died elderly at half the age of most sheep (6 years).[161]

Thus far (December 31, 2018), there has not been a cloned human and they are not likely to occur. Researchers are interested in embryonic stem cell cloning for therapeutic reasons, to replace damaged tissue, but there is a great risk of cancer. In a moment, we will address current optimistic adult alternatives in embryonic stem cell research.

Ethical Issues of Cloning

Before considering stem cell research, it is useful to look at some of the ethical issues of cloning provided by the NIH fact sheet.

> Reproductive cloning would present the potential of creating a human that is genetically identical to another person who has previously existed or who still exists. This may conflict with long-standing religious and societal values about human dignity, possibly infringing upon principles of individual freedom, identity and autonomy. However, some argue that reproductive cloning could help sterile couples fulfill their dream of parenthood. Others see human cloning as a way to avoid passing on a deleterious gene that runs in the family without having to undergo embryo screening or embryo selection.[162]

The person's freedom, identity, and autonomy referred to in the quote, is the new individual with a cloned origin. He or she would not be a unique individual; their genetic identity would be almost fully known as expressed by the originating person. Dolly's rapid aging casts a deep

[159] "Cloning," p.4.

[160] https://www.genome.gov/25020028/cloning-fact-sheet/

[161] http://www.cnn.com/2003/WORLD/europe/02/14/cloned.dolly.dies/ (accessed January 17, 2015).

[162] See note 158.

shadow on human cloning.

Stem Cell Research

The following content is summarized from a fact sheet provided by Bedford Stem Cell Research Foundation, Frequently Asked Questions.[163] A **stem cell** is a reserve cell available to grow and repair tissues like the skin. There are also stem cells in the liver and fatty tissues. For some tissues there are no cells on reserve in the body tissues to self-repair. These include the heart, spinal cord, brain and pancreas. If there were stem cells available these could provide potential repair for many ailments like Parkinson's disease, diabetes and spinal cord severance. Embryonic stem cells are pluripotent and can become any cell in the body. The difficulty with adult stem cells is their very limited capacity to become different body cells. But from Bedford, we find that the use of embryonic stem cells has two physiologic drawbacks, the cells can become cancerous as we said before, but they are also subject to rejection as foreign to the body of the recipient. In addition, there is serious moral concern about using an embryo to heal an adult, the embryo dies when the stem cells are removed. This would mean that a vulnerable class of humans is sacrificed for another more established class of humans.

For these philosophical and ethical concerns, Bedford and other research associations are now using the individual's own stem cells to provide tissue for healing. According to Bedford Research Foundation, there are now three types of pluripotent stem cells:

1) **Embryonic stem cells from fertilized eggs** are good models for research, but they have ethical issues, and will have tissue rejection problems (similar to bone marrow and kidney transplants).

2) **Parthenote stem cells (derived from *un*fertilized eggs, "activated eggs")** may be as pluripotent as embryonic stem cells, and have been the focus of BSCRF (Bedford) scientists for several years. Studies using monkey parthenote stem cells to treat Parkinson's disease have been very promising.

   • Parthenotes do not have the potential tissue rejection problems faced by stem cells derived from fertilized eggs.

---

[163] http://www.bedfordresearch.org/stemcell/stemcell.php?item=what-is-a-stem-cell (Last accessed December 31, 2018).

- Unlike adult stem cells, parthenotes can potentially become any cell in the body. They are also less controversial than stem cells that are derived from fertilized eggs.
3) **Induced Pluripotent stem cells** are derived by adding proteins that reprogram adult cells, reverting them to their embryonic state. "These new cells are expected to live for a very long time while retaining the ability to form all of the different tissues found in a human body.[164]

Parents can reserve frozen cord blood from their child for potential future need. Cord blood cells are not pluripotent but multipotent. They can give rise to all the cells in normal bone marrow. This is very good news for parents as leukemia is such a threat to children.

Parthenote stem cells are now available from testes and ova of women of child bearing age. These Pluripotent stem cells are from stimulation and growth of cells into the needed tissues. Since these tissues are from the individual in need there is no tissue rejection. There are also reports of induced pluripotent stem cell therapies being developed that do not involve fertilized eggs and are available to people of different ages, gender, and racial groups. These cells do not destabilize towards cancer or trigger rejection as embryonic cells do. These alternatives offer promising therapies for the future.

Conclusion

Our concern in this chapter has been moral and ethical issues related to human generation. While we have proposed the granting of protected rights based on one's humanity, this perspective has had a long and difficult history. The Declaration of Independence does not use person, it uses the term "men," and it secures the rights of "life, liberty, and the pursuit of happiness" based on our created humanity. We are aware that in plantation America the framers of our Declaration of Independence and our Constitution addressed only male citizens and many of its framers supported slavery. It was another 100 years before the Emancipation Proclamation. Legally secured rights for all regardless of age (from birth), race, gender, or disability were secured in the middle of the Twentieth Century taking another 50 years and massive demonstrations.

There is an interesting passage about humanity within the Constitution reads:

---

[164] See n.161.

> While it is important to realize the government does not fulfill the rights but does not interfere with them, for our purposes, we note that these rights pre-exist the Constitution. It is generally considered that they reside within the being of citizens, within their humanity.[165]

In 1993, I was teaching an evening ethics class for adult students. Distinctions were made in the topic of abortion provided by the language itself, mother versus woman and baby versus fetus. I decided to share what I had recently learned at a lecture by the famous cyrogeneticist (study of frozen genetic content), Jerome Lejeune,[166] who discovered the chromosomal anomaly for Downs Syndrome. I described his discussion of the roles male and female gametes play in the generation of a new human. It was really interesting because he was speaking from his own research (on mice). If two ova were stimulated to unite chromosomes and begin cellular development (parthenogenesis) the result is the body of the fetus. If two male nuclei are united they produce placental and amniotic sac tissues. He was answering the question if same sex partners could have their own children and pointed to the differences between male and female functions and how the generation of new life requires both. As he put it women are all about taking care of the body and men are about providing food and shelter.

Lejeune also made the point that molecular embryos are distinct in appearance, even at the one cell stage, the zygote. He said if a student could not tell the difference between a human zygote and an ape zygote they would fail his class.

My presentation was animated because I felt excited about this scientific approach to the discussion of human life and of how clear and humorous his lecture was. The class was attended by approximately fifteen adult business students. A student about five chairs in front of me blurted loudly, "I don't care. I'm going to do what I'm going to do, if I want to." Even if the little one is human, I queried. "That's right," she said. I called a break, erased the board, and collected myself. It is always one of my goals to avoid the rancor that can enter abortion debates. My position is and was that people need accurate information so they can make good decisions.

Sometimes emotion overrules reason. Emotion may substitute for reason. There are many who have had to have an abortion, as they saw the situation. We know women died from self-induced or back alley abortions for hundreds, even thousands of years. It used to be the case that if you

---

[165] http://www.usconstitution.net/consttop_resp.html
[166] Michael J. Mcgivney Lecture, Providence Hospital, Washington, D.C.

were unmarried and pregnant, you would be shunned by your community. I recall as a child the girl across the street left town and returned several months later with a baby. The father supposedly died before the baby was born. When trapped by an unwanted, feared pregnancy, women search for a solution. What could be a precious child becomes a problem, a mistake.

Women make the best decision they can within their difficult circumstances. A woman needs support. Support can make all the difference in one's mental and physical health regardless of the decision made. The language of choice is avoided because choices narrow and one's ability to think is blurred with the fear and stress experienced. But we know the unborn is a living human that will probably actualize its potential to be a living baby if left in the womb.

It has been the position of this book that one's view of human life stands behind what is seen as an issue in personal and professional ethics, what generates an ethical dilemma; and what resolves it. For this reason, after considering values and their impact in our lives, we began with a classical perspective of human life as substantial and relational.

Conversation Starters:

1. Hospitals do so much to enrich human life and to bring health and comfort to people. Laboratory personnel, x-ray technicians, respiratory therapists and health record librarians certainly do not participate in surgical procedures, but if there were a moral concern with some procedures would there be any moral accountability for the above staff in supporting the institution itself?

2. Thomas Jefferson penned the words "all men are created equal "and he meant "men "as women and children were like property. As a plantation owner in Virginia, he found no contradiction owning slaves as property. Slaves were considered less than human, almost but not human. Can you think of examples today where individuals are treated as less than human and as such, their right to life, liberty, and the pursuit of happiness is threatened?

3. In an analogy, some aspects are the same and some different. Gazzaniga's analogy says, if Home Depot burnt down no homes would be lost, only supplies. In the same way, humans are only potential persons. Humans can be lost or destroyed without losing persons. What are the aspects that match, what are the differences? Is this analogy clarifying? Does this analogy hold? If anything is missing, what is it?

4. What about the little one changes at birth that provides the right to life? Given that the fetus can be legally killed, even in the birth canal, this seems to be the moment of acquiring rights. Support your answers with premises from science and reason.

5. What ethical concerns emerge with the freezing or discarding of unused embryos? If you could ensure the fertilized embryos were all implanted and brought to birth, would there still be concerns with IVF?

6. Reason to an answer for the following with the Principle of Double Effect as your standard:

a. Unmarried and pregnant, you will be killed by your community. Is an abortion warranted?

b. You are pregnant near the end of your fifth month, your organs are shutting down. You are told you will die in a few days if your pregnancy is continued. Is an abortion warranted?

c. You are about to graduate from high school and you have college scholarships when you discover you are pregnant. Is an abortion warranted?

Reflection Submissions:
Thoughtfulness, not a particular position, is expected. Support your answers.

1. If one were to decide abortions are morally wrong, does performing abortions nullify all the other good done by the medical facility?
2. It seems clear that the founders of our country were referring to a divine creator. In what ways, if at all, does contemporary negation of God impact the Declaration of Independence statement grounding moral rights and leading to passage of civil rights? Supposing there is no God, what is required for society to respect and care for all citizens? Support your answers.
3. This is a good time for you to assert a position when human life begins and when moral rights are attributed to the new individual, include rationales for your position. What difference does it make? Write your thoughts on each of the following: Would your view on abortion, cloning, or embryonic stem cell research change given each of the following possibilities?
    a. What if there is no immaterial soul, the mind is an expression of biochemical function, sometimes called epiphenomena?
    b. What if the individual is an expression of the evolutionary process?
    c. What if the individual comes into existence with a soul from an ultimate immaterial source?
    d. What if an ultimate being did design the universe but has no further involvement in human life?

Outline for Chapter 9: Ethical Issues Related to the Beginning of Life
A. Moral and Legal Accountability
   1. Personal experience
   2. An experience of Socrates
   3. Iimplied consent
B. Acquiring Protection of Human Rights
   1. When life begins
   2. Defining life
   3. Personhood
   4. Symmetry between the beginning of life and the declaration of death
     a. Cardiac declaration of death
     b. Whole-brain criteria of death
     c. Higher brain death as a criterion
   5. The informed decision

C. Impact of Technology
  1. In-vitro fertilization (IVF)
    a. Moral considerations of IVF include financial and human costs
  2. Cloning
    a. Ethical issues of cloning
  3. Stem Cell Research
D. Conclusion

Terminology for Chapter 9
Self-defense argument
Principle of double effect
Hominization
Individuation
Rationality
Stem cell
Implied Consent
Cardiac declaration of death
Whole-brain death
Higher brain death
Human genome

CHAPTER 10

ISSUES AT THE END OF LIFE

Objectives

This chapter provides an opportunity for you to:

1. Describe how brain death occurs from anoxia and from severe head trauma.
2. Describe the impact of clinical and brain death parameters on organ retrieval and transplantation with the dead donor rule.
3. Describe when patients and families ought to omit CPR.
4. Compare and contrast each of the following end of life distinctions: active and passive euthanasia, ordinary and extraordinary care, killing versus letting die, natural versus artificial interventions, and palliative versus futile care.
5. Use the principle of double effect and its criteria for end of life decisions.
6. Evaluate your proposed positions on issues at the end of life.

Parameters for Declaring Death

At this time, health-care technology makes it possible to maintain the tissues of the body while the brain is no longer functioning. This is very helpful in preserving organs for retrieval and transplantation into needy recipients. Nonetheless, it is very confusing for families of the deceased person. They are told their loved one is dead when they can see him or her breathe; even though it is ventilator assisted, their body is warm and they have a pulse. You can sense their bewilderment, "What do you mean he is dead?"

Clinical Death

The average person holds the loss of respiration and circulation as death. This is called **clinical death. Brain death** is counter intuitive and requires much explanation for the person who only knows clinical death as death. This is a significant issue because organ donation and retrieval require a dead donor. By the time clinical death occurs most organs have deteriorated significantly and cannot be used for transplantation. Great care is taken to treat and restore the injured person. Organ donation becomes a possibility only after it is believed the patient cannot live.

Brain Death

The brain is the integrating organ for the energizing principle of life, the form or soul. Since 1968, brain death has been confirmed by the **Harvard criteria**. There has not been a recorded return to functioning once brain death has been accurately established. Although some scholars and physicians do not accept the Harvard criteria of brain death, in all 50 states, brain death is accepted as death.[167] The following are the assessment parameters of the Harvard Brain Death Criteria: (1) condition has a known cause, (2) condition is irreversible, (3) neuromuscular blocking agents and central nervous system depressants are absent, (4) temperature is higher than 35°C (95°F), (5) patient is apneic (not breathing), (6) patient is areflexic (not showing reflex responses).[168]

A Case of Brain Death Following Cerebral Anoxia

The introductory chapter noted that in December, 2013, the BBC posted headlines following a California court decision to extend life support another week for Jahi McMath. The 13-year-old girl hemorrhaged after tonsillectomy surgery and went into cardiac arrest. She was placed on a ventilator for life support, and then three days later she was assessed as brain dead.[169] Brain death is the natural outcome from a lack of oxygen to

---

[167] James L. Bernat, Charles M. Culver, and Bernard Gert, in "Defining Death in Theory and Practice,"
http://www2.sunysuffolk.edu/pecorip/SCCCWEB/ETEXTS/DeathandDying_TEXT/Bernat_Culver_Gert.htm (accessed August 30, 2013).
[168] Ad Hoc Committee of the Harvard Medical School to Examine the Definition of Brain Death. JAMA 1968;205(6):337–40; The Quality Standards Subcommittee of the American Academy of Neurology. Neurology 1995;45(5):1012–4. A more contemporary and detailed account of establishing brain death can be found at the following site: American Academy of Neurology Guidelines for Brain Death Determination. http://surgery.med.miami.edu/laora/clinical-operations/brain-death-diagnosis (accessed July 15, 2018).
[169] (December 30) http://www.bbc.co.uk/news/world-us-canada-25552818

the brain, cerebral anoxia. It is quite reasonable for her family to have thought of her as alive. They saw her chest rise and fall with ventilation. Cardiac rhythm was restored so the body had warmth. However, for one who is brain dead, there is no detectable brain activity.

From the beginning of health-care records, death was identified as having occurred when the heart stopped and one stopped breathing. Brain death by the Harvard Criteria is fairly new; just since 1968.

Moral and Ethical Considerations of this Case

By the principle of non-contradiction, one cannot be both dead and alive. Thinking about our earlier discussions of what it is to be human, we can say that the body on the ventilator was Jahi's body, but was it Jahi? If Plato and Descartes are right that the soul dwells in the body, the soul could have left. If Aristotle was right that humans are matter-form unities, when the metabolizing human materials are present the animating form or soul is also present. In this perspective, Jahi was her matter-form unity in the bed. If the brain is the integrating organ of the body and the brain is not functioning, for Aristotle, her soul may be present but unable to express its human function of conscious thought. It could be the ventilator is inhibiting the natural progression to death. Even so, the ethical standard of 'doing no harm' would seem to ask us to keep her on the ventilator as this is less harmful since death is irreversible. But is keeping her on the ventilator doing 'the good'? Keeping the girl on the ventilator respects the mother's wishes for her child and one can presume a thirteen-year-old would seek to live at all costs. But, preventing her death, when she cannot live, is not a human good.

Confronting Reality

The family considered her alive, but it is a mistake to think either a court order or the family's desire means she is alive. Neither does having a death certificate mean Jahi is dead. She had a death certificate from the state of California since December 2013. Conversely, not having a death certificate would not mean she was alive. Documentation needs to reflect reality; it does not make reality.

(accessed January 1, 2014.

Personal Moral Decisions

Jahi was removed from the hospital in California and never taken off of the ventilator. Two and a half years later, Jahi's mother sought to have the death certificate voided.[170] The death certificate impacted the opportunities available for her care. Jahi was taken to New Jersey because their legal system enabled her mother's religious objection to removal of the ventilator to override the death certificate. Cardiac, clinical death is the only acceptable criteria for some religions and cultures.

Health-care Funding

There is some question whether keeping Jahi alive was the best use of Medicaid funds, but this is a persistent question in the allocation of scarce resources. The principle of justice questions the use of health-care funds, but there were pro-life groups who assisted with expenses. This is how they wanted to use their money, even though it could be argued there were better ways to spend it. On June 22nd 2018, Jahi experienced clinical death, the irreversible stoppage of her heart following surgery for an intestinal issue.[171]

Practice Concerns

During the years of Jahi's care in her New Jersey apartment, the primary decision to be made by health-care professionals was whether or not in good conscience they could work within this situation. As a practitioner, my personal goal in this complex situation would be to not increase the family's burden. If the ventilator is keeping her clinically alive, removal of this life support may be seen as killing her. This could lead to the conclusion that removal of life support killed her when she was already dead or dying in a process that was interrupted. Removal of the ventilator would be letting her die. This recalls the concerns of health-care providers in Karen Ann Quinlan's case discussed in Chapter Four.

---

[170] http://blackdoctor.org/484482/family-of-jahi-mcmath-say-she-is-healthy-as-beautiful-as-ever/2/

[171] http://www.latimes.com/local/lanow/la-me-ln-jahi-mcmath-dies-20180628-story.html

Brain Death after Severe Head Trauma

Jahi more than likely suffered cerebral anoxia, a diffuse lack of oxygen to the brain from circulatory failure. Another common cause of brain death is head trauma with resulting swelling and compression forcing the brain into the spinal canal through the foramen magnum.

The following account by the ICU nurse Kathleen Peiffer describes how brain death occurs after severe head trauma:

> The initial trauma sets off a cascade of events. Tissue damage and fluid blockage or excessive fluid accumulation result in increasing intracranial pressure, ischemia, and brain cell death. When ischemia reaches the brain stem, it triggers a massive release of catecholamines—an event known as an autonomic or sympathetic "storm"—which leads to an immediate, intense Cushing response (increased systemic vascular resistance and hypertension) lasting about 15 minutes. Compression of the vasculature and worsening ischemia cause infarction of brain tissue. Venous engorgement and brain swelling cause the brain to herniate through the foramen magnum, further inhibiting cerebral perfusion. Inflammation and edema progress and intracranial pressure rises even more, culminating in a complete loss of cerebral blood flow.[172]

Normally, the skull protects the brain. It is a tight box, a shell, that stabilizes the delicate brain tissues, but there is very little extra room. Bleeding and swelling are normal responses to injury whether you hit your arm or your head, but the fluids in the skull have no place to go and tissues cannot expand resulting in compression of the brain.

When Brain Death Does Not Occur

Anoxia and severe trauma both result in brain death, but when injury is not so severe that brain death occurs, the edema will begin to recede in about two weeks. Specific medications are given that reduce edema in the brain to assist in this reduction of intracranial pressure. Because of the possibility of recovered function, some practitioners recommend keeping the person on the ventilator for a period of time to see if function will be restored. When the brain stem still functions, but there is a disconnect between the body and higher brain functions, there is usually a diagnosis of persistent or permanent vegetative state (PVS). If there is a lack of

---

[172] Kathleen M.Z. Peiffer, *American Journal of Nursing*, March 2007, pp. 58-67. http://www.nursingcenter.com/prodev/cearticleprint.asp?CE_ID=698333 (accessed on line Mar.18, 2009).

communication between hemispheres of the brain and the spinal nerves, the diagnosis is locked-in syndrome. A loss of consciousness with **coma** may occur from any number of life traumas. This coma may transition to a restoration of consciousness or a persistent vegetative state.

The Practitioner's Role

As health-care providers, we have a moral obligation to provide accurate information in answering questions or making suggestions. Families cling to any shred of hope. Providing factual information about the patient's condition from within the current situation is better than assertions about the future that may lead to false hope. It is wise for practitioners to be cautious and not express beyond what is known and the practice expectations of their disciplines.

Judicial Intervention

For the judge to assert a court order to keep Jahi alive on the ventilator, as reported in December 2013, was to say that she was alive, which would have been false if the brain death diagnosis was accurate. This situation was tragic, and the family needed time to accept the reality of her death. The judge was probably keeping her on the ventilator for her family. This is common with sudden serious injuries. In the case of Jahi, she did remain on the ventilator for five years. Her mother asserts she physiologically went through puberty while on the ventilator. Usually, the brain is seen as coordinating organ for these bodily developments.

A Word of Caution

These distinctions are being noted because, as stated in chapter nine, good moral decisions require accurate knowledge of bodily states and knowledge of particular clinical circumstances. With accurate information one can better consider ethical actions. Matters of treatment orders following diagnosis of brain dysfunction are not within the domain of non-medical practice. But many times, staff members will engage in discussion without understanding the diagnosis. This information may have resolved their perceived ethical tensions. Families turn to health-care providers for guidance. The critical moral requirement is to not provide misinformation or encourage false hope.

Active and Passive Euthanasia

The overwhelming majority of those dying are dying from terminal illness, dementia, and aging. It is clear that death is inevitable. Given the natural course of events as we know them, none of us will avoid death. The only real position is acceptance of death. This acceptance allows you to focus on interventions that promote quality living and do not stand in the way of peaceful dying.

There is an important distinction between active and passive euthanasia. **Active euthanasia** is an intervention that kills. **Passive euthanasia** is letting the person die. This may be not starting or the removal of life prolonging interventions, like the ventilator. You will remember from previous chapters the assertion that all life is worth living, but not all interventions are worth having. Facing the reality of death, those who are dying may consider the difference between taking their own life by suicide or assisted suicide; or dying because interventions were rejected. These questions are serious as we want to promote health and not kill, while not interfering with the natural process of dying.

Nutrition and Hydration

For Organ Donors

With the definitive diagnosis of brain death, food and fluids are only provided if the individual will be an organ donor. According to Peiffer, "If interventions after brain death are not aggressive and timely, the body's tissues and organs cannot be used for transplantation. Indeed, when a patient is a potential or designated organ donor, the nursing care required may be even more rigorous after brain death than before... (She adds, at my facility, the nurse-patient ratio for brain-dead organ donors may be as high as 3:1). She continues, "The brain is in charge of the proper functioning of all body systems. In a patient who is brain dead, therefore, keeping the donor organs viable involves, in a sense, fooling the body into thinking the brain is still functioning." [173] Thus, to maintain metabolic activity for viability of the organs, nutrition and hydration will be continued but there is not a sense of keeping the patient alive.

Neurological Deficits

With persistent or permanent vegetative states, locked-in syndrome, minimal brain function, dementias and terminal illnesses the moral question of whether or not to provide food and fluids becomes acutely

---

[173] Ibid.

relevant. The three young ladies (Karen Quinlan, Nancy Cruzan, and Terry Schiavo) whose landmark court decisions led to the withdrawal of interventions to allow the patient to die when they were afflicted with permanent vegetative states were all Catholic. Because of this, Robert Fine provides the two competing Catholic "viewpoints on the morality of withholding or withdrawing ANH (artificial nutrition and hydration)."[174] The view promoted by Pope John Paul II in 2004 is that ANH is "obligatory and must be maintained in most cases of persistent vegetative state.[175] Fine holds that the Pope's position is fatally flawed by a misunderstanding of the permanence of the clinical state of one considered to be permanently vegetative. This is hard to support because the Pope's position derives from ANH being one way to provide for the ordinary care of nutrition and hydration. It is not tied to the permanence or temporary status of the condition. Additionally, Fine asserts it is impossible for this individual to suffer because of the disconnect between sensation and higher brain capacities. He holds that one must be conscious to suffer.[176] Pope John Paul II asserts we do not know for sure the person cannot suffer. "Moreover, it is not possible to rule out *a priori* that the withdrawal of nutrition and hydration, as reported by authoritative studies, is the source of considerable suffering for the sick person, even if we can see only the reactions at the level of the autonomic nervous system (that is, reflexive) or of gestures. Modern clinical neurophysiology and neuro-imaging techniques, in fact, seem to point to the lasting quality in these patients of elementary forms of communication and analysis of stimuli."[177] Fine will go on to say that ANH cannot be nourishment that alleviates suffering because, again, these patients cannot suffer. Fine does note respect for individuals in the image of a creative designer, but he invokes this as a reason to not keep them alive in an incapacitated state when Pope John Paul II uses this to call health-care personnel to value and preserve all human life. The Pope writes "However, it is not enough to reaffirm the general principle according to which the value of a man's life cannot be made subordinate to any judgment of its quality expressed by other men; it is necessary to promote the *taking of positive actions* as a stand against

---

[174] Robert L. Fine, From Quinlan to Schiavo: medical ethical, and legal issues in severe brain injury. *BUMC Proceedings* 2005; 18:303-310.), P. 308-309.

[175] Pope John Paul II. Care for patients in a 'permanent vegetative state.' Origins 2004;33(43):737,739-740. Also available http://www.vatican.va/holy_father/john_paul_ii/speeches/2004/march/documents/h f_jp-ii_spe_20040320_congress-fiamc_en.html. (Last accessed January 4, 2019).

[176] Fine, p. 303.

[177] Pope, paragraph 5.

pressures to withdraw hydration and nutrition as a way to put an end to the lives of these patients."[178]

Fine writes that "The view that ANH is morally optional and may be withdrawn in most cases of persistent vegetative state was common in much of Catholic thinking prior to March 2004 (the date of Pope John Paul II"s address) "[179] This older view is grounded on the dualistic notion that the spiritual life is more important that the physical life of the body. (This recalls Plato's dualism.) Pope John Paul II is well known for his promotion of the unity of body and soul and the sacredness of the body. (We think of Aristotle's preference for the unity of body and soul.) This would be the source of critical differences in positions of Fine and Pope John Paul II. In 1957, Pope Pius the XII wrote, "Life, health, all temporal activities are in fact subordinated to spiritual ends."[180] In 2004, the respected Catholic ethicist, Fr. Kevin O'Rourke argued, ANH is "not only futile, because it is ineffective in helping the patient pursue the higher goals of life, but is excessively burdensome because it maintains persistent vegetative state patients in a condition in which this pursuit [of higher goals] will never again be possible."[181] Fine writes, "Many devoutly religious persons have told me during my medical practice that they prefer a life in heaven to a life in a profoundly brain-injured state."[182] The moral struggle is to resolve if withholding food and fluid is setting up an internal environment so that the person will die (killing) or if it is just letting them die.

Enhancing Life or Preventing Death

As you can see, from this discussion, there is no "cut and dry," definitive answer. Some of the most difficult decisions made by patients, families, and practitioners are made at the end of a person's life. With the change from paternalistic care to autonomy more of the decision-making falls to the patient and his or her family. At an ethics discussion at a nearby hospital a young ethicist, Valerie Satkoske, said something startling. She asked how many of us believed in life after death. Almost all of us raised our hands. Shockingly, she then said, "Why do you not act like it?" She continued, "You keep everyone alive on this earth as long as

---

[178] Pope, paragraph 6.

[179] Fine, p.308.

[180] Pope Pius XII. The prolongation of life (November 24, 1957). *The Pope Speaks* 1958; 4(4):395-396. Reprinted in *Origins* 2004;33 (43). In Fine, p. 309

[181] O'Rourke K. *Origins* 2004;33(43):746. In Fine, p. 309.

[182] Fine, p.309.

you possibly can. With all of these unconscious patients, are you preserving and enhancing life or preventing death?"[183]

In the preceding section, Fine made the same challenge as Satkoske did. In Fine's discussion of justice in funding, he concludes, "I believe there is a very cogent argument in favor of supporting patients who can experience joy in life rather than those who are merely vegetating and cannot experience any joy in life."[184] Many Christians, especially Catholics, embrace the Natural Law position that we ought to preserve life even if there is dementia or coma. I would propose the need to feed everyone comes from this principle. When one does not eat, they surely die. This is definitive. This is difficult, but worthy of further thought.

Withholding Food and Fluids

For consideration of provision or withholding food and fluids at the end of prolonged illness, we turn to a publication of the National Cancer Institute, at the National Institutes of Health. They have an on-line publication called, "The Last Days of Life (PDQ)."[185] These comments are taken from the Health Professional Version.

> The controversial nature of providing artificial nutrition at the end of life has prompted the American Academy of Hospice and Palliative Medicine (AAHPM) to recommend that individual clinical situations be assessed using clinical judgment and skill to determine when artificial nutrition is appropriate. Recognizing that the primary intention of nutrition is to benefit the patient, AAHPM concludes that withholding artificial nutrition near the end of life may be appropriate medical care if the risks outweigh the possible benefit to the patient.
>
> The goal of end-of-life care is to relieve suffering and alleviate distressing symptoms (goals of palliative care). The patient's needs and desires must be the focus, with their best interests being the guide for decision making, influenced by religious, ethical, and compassionate issues (parenthetical content added) (Section: Nutritional Supplementation).[186]

---

[183] Valerie Satkoske, "Ethics and Humanities", conference at Wheeling Hospital, 2011.

[184] Fine, p.310.

[185] http://www.cancer.gov/cancertopics/pdq/supportivecare/lasthours/health professional/page2/AllPages/Print

[186] Ibid.

Hard Choices for Loving People

Some years ago (2001), Chaplain Hank Dunn authored *Hard Choices for Loving People: CPR, Artificial Feeding, Comfort Care, and the Patient with a Life-Threatening Illness*. His goal was to "provide guidance to patients and their families who must face the 'hard choices' as they receive and participate in health care."[187] He identifies four of the critical questions impacting end of life treatment decisions. One's moral beliefs determine how you answer these questions, and they are important questions for to be answered. The identified questions are: (1) Shall resuscitation be attempted? (2) Shall artificial nutrition and hydration be utilized? (3) Should a nursing home resident or someone ill at home be hospitalized? (4) Is it time to shift the treatment goal from cure to hospice or comfort care only? Underneath these questions is the haunting question, "Is human life to be preserved at all costs?"

If you answer, "Yes, it is never right to let a person die," these questions disappear and you do not sign the Do Not Resuscitate order, withdraw or withhold food and fluids, transfer care to hospice or comfort care only, and you do transfer all persons to the hospital for aggressive treatment.

If you say, "No, there are times when we need to let go of medical interventions and let nature take its course. Let the individual die." Then we must determine when this time has arrived. This is not asking if health care providers ought to participate in an individual's death by actions intended to kill. But, the question is when is it right to withhold intervention(s) and let them die. The reasonable, virtuous person may hold that every life is worth living, but some interventions are not worth having.

Mutual Goal Setting for Supporting Families

In terms of a specific patient situation, one must evaluate the potential outcomes or goals for this particular patient and the possible benefit (s) of this particular intervention. Goals could include cure, stabilization, or preparation for a peaceful death. Stabilization could mean restoration or it may mean life at a lower level of function. Patients and families need to decide what level of expected function is required for them to accept aggressive treatments and when they only want comfort or palliative interventions. Within patient care, outcomes are only probable, but patients and families need to be aware of expected probable results from

---

[187] Herndon, Virginia: A&A Publishers, Inc., 2001. p. 6.

interventions. Most often this information needs to be provided by the physician, but other professionals can reinforce instructions and assist families in framing helpful questions. The best decisions are made with clear and accurate information, but one needs to stay within the practice parameters of their discipline and direct medical practice questions to physicians. From your class that included communications, you will recall the importance of deflecting questions back to the patient or family saying, what do you think? Or, what are your concerns?

With providing food and fluids to incapacitated patients the critical question is whether the intervention is beneficial to the patient or doing harm. Theoretically we can discuss whether medical feeding and fluid provision is natural or artificial, but what could be more natural than receiving or providing food and fluids for our continued existence. From birth, receiving nourishment has been a community event. Without someone to feed the little child, the child dies. An elderly or disabled person will also die if not provided food and fluids.

Comfort Care Feeding

The issue is not whether to spoon feed, or instill formula through a tube; the question is whether or not this food and this fluid are helpful or harmful at this time. The answer is found in careful assessment of patient responses to food. With the additional fluid, is the patient nourished or pushed into fluid overload with back up into the lungs and extremities. Both spoon feeding and tube feeding can lead to aspiration pneumonia.

Spoon feeding is preferable to many health practitioners and families because of the required social interaction and it is more natural to eat from utensils. In long term care facilities, social interaction is a goal, the desirable standard. Nonetheless, two paid staff certified in feeding and working in the same room can easily be talking to each other rather than the nursing home residents. Additionally, with several patients to feed, nursing assistances are happy to have residents indicate they want no more, no matter how little they have eaten. It is much faster to hang tube feeding, but lying in bed with liquid running into your stomach or small intestine through a tube challenges the meaning of having a meal. This image represents the negative meaning of artificial nutrition. But, for some people tube feeding is just right.

Working as a visiting nurse some years ago, I met patients living with tube feedings and parenteral hyper-alimentation. One day I visited a lady at her home to check her abdominal site which had eroded and looked infected. Because of surgery for esophageal cancer she could not eat orally, but she could visit neighbors, watch T.V., shop, and enjoy her family. She received strength from the liquid feedings that allowed her to do activities she wanted to do. Clearly, she was not terminal. The point is just that artificial feeding through a tube can be the right intervention for some people.

The Last Days

According to Dunn, when the illness gets to the terminal stage in the last few days of life, our bodies do not digest the food eaten either by mouth or feeding tube. The undigested food can cause bloating, discomfort and regurgitation with possible aspiration. In this case, not feeding makes really good sense falling within the maxim "first do no harm." Sometimes, feeding can lead to harm.[188] It seems counter-intuitive but Dunn writes, "The medical evidence is quite clear that dehydration in the end stage of a terminal illness is a very natural and compassionate way to die."[189] One wonders how this can be, but Dunn reports there is a natural release of pain-relieving chemicals as the body dehydrates and the physiological state that comes with no food intake suppresses appetite and causes a sense of well-being. He concludes the point, "No matter what the treatment choice regarding feeding tubes, comfort care and freedom from pain are essential goals of any medical team."[190] It is important to realize this care at the end stage of a terminal illness does not include someone in a persistent vegetative state, or dementia. This end stage is when the dying individual enters their final few days. The body systems are actively shutting down in the natural process of death.

Dunn provides the benefits of not using artificial hydration (for example, an IV or feeding tube) in a dying patient. These include: (1) less fluid in the lungs and therefore, less congestion, making breathing easier;(2) less fluid in the throat and, therefore, less need for suctioning;(3) less pressure around tumors and, therefore, less pain; (4) and less urination and, therefore, less need to move the patient for changing the bed and less risk of bedsores;(5) a natural release of pain-relieving chemicals as the body dehydrates. According to Dunn, some have even described it as 'mild euphoria.' This state that comes with no food intake also suppresses appetite and causes a sense of well-being. Dunn concludes, "The medical evidence is quite clear that dehydration in the end stage of a terminal

---

[188] Dunn, p.21.
[189] Dunn, p.22.
[190] Dunn, p.23.

illness is a very natural and compassionate way to die."[191]

Resuscitation

According to the report of the National Cancer Institute, "Broadly defined, resuscitation includes all interventions that provide cardiovascular, respiratory, and metabolic support necessary to maintain and sustain the life of a dying patient (section on Resuscitation)." [192]The report cautions, "It is important for patients, families, and proxies to understand that choices may be made specifying what supportive measures, if any, should be given preceding death and at the time of death."[193] This information must be determined prior to the moment of death. Without a written document, interventions may be begun that may make the final minutes of one's life more burdensome. If a DNR (Do Not Resuscitate) order is not in place, staff at the hospital are obliged by law and policy to begin CPR (Cardio Pulmonary Resuscitation). And, as Dunn says there is not a little CPR. If the patient is at home and 911 is called the first responders are obliged by law to do everything possible to save the person's life, unless there is an accessible and valid form for DNR or DNH (Do Not Hospitalize), or DNT (Do Not Transport). If your patient and their family want the patient to die in peace at home, instruct them to not call 911. With this call they will likely be transported to the hospital for aggressive treatment. If your patient and their family want the patient to die at home prepare the necessary documents and make arrangements with the funeral home. Morticians are familiar with the process and with prior arrangements they can be called after the person dies to pick up the body. Dunn provides a critical realization: "CPR severely reduces the possibility of a peaceful death."[194] Many families do make arrangements to have the patient die at home and then call 911. But, it is frightening to watch someone struggle for breath. The family may find themselves unable to do this. If all of the paperwork is in place, first responders can transport the person and they can be admitted to a medical bed for the last days or hours of life. This final distress of the patient and family can be markedly reduced by working with Hospice.

---

[191] Dunn, p. 22, 23.
[192] https://www.cancer.gov/publications/dictionaries/cancer-terms/def/cardiopulmonary-resuscitation(accessed January 1, 2019).
[193] See n.173.
[194] Dunn, p.14.

Value and Concerns

At this point, we would do well to take a closer look at the value and concerns of resuscitation efforts at the end of life. Dunn reports a review of 113 studies of the use of CPR in hospitals over a 33 year period. Resuscitation was attempted on 35% of hospital patients and 3% of nursing home residents whose heart had stopped. Significantly of "26,095 patients who received resuscitation attempts, 3968 or 15.2 percent survived to be discharged from the hospital."[195] Generally healthy patients with an abnormal heart rhythm (ventricular tachycardia or fibrillation) were most likely to survive to be discharged (21 %). Patients with the least chance of survival and discharge (less than 2%) had more than one or two medical problems, were dependent on others for their care, or had "advanced, irreparable organ failures."[196]

Dunn asks "Why does CPR offer so little hope of medical benefit for the frail, debilitated nursing home resident? Most of the characteristics that point to a poor prognosis for the survival of hospital patients are common in nursing home residents."[197] Some nursing homes have a no CPR policy for their center; staff call 911 if the patient collapses and there is no plan in place for the patient to die at the nursing home. Family and resident would have to transfer to another home if CPR is desired. Given the poor outcomes, it seems CPR is not warranted for this population. In fact, CPR would be doing harm to a resident. This does not mean that acute illness will not be treated. The person can still be transported to the hospital for evaluation and care. What this means is if the heart stops, the staff will not act to restart it. To perform CPR is to provide futile care.

Comfort Care and Letting Die

Many people struggle with stopping an intervention that was started, even if the intervention is not doing any good and may, in fact, be causing difficulty for the patient and family. Rather than seeing this removal of the intervention as an opportunity to stop doing harm, some people think that stopping what seems to be a life promoting intervention, even if ineffective, is killing by omission. They are missing the distinction between killing and letting die. Sometimes the kindest thing to do is to

---

[195] Dunn, p.12.
[196] Saklayen, Mohammad, Liss, Howard, and Markert, Ronald. In-hospital cardiopulmonary resuscitation: Survival in 1 hospital and Literature Review, Medicine, 74: 163-175, 1995. In Dunn, p. 12.
[197] Dunn, p.13.

stop an intervention and let the patient die. The intervention is standing in the way of a natural sequence of events. Stopping nutrition and hydration because it is causing fluids to build up and harming the patient is very different from stopping nutrition and hydration so that the patient will die.

The difference between stopping a ventilator and stopping artificial nutrition and hydration is that food and fluids must be brought to each and every one of us. Medical nutrition and hydration is just another way of providing what nature requires. If a ventilator is discontinued, the patient still has the opportunity to receive oxygen from the ambient air, as was the case when Karen Quinlan's ventilator was removed. The alternative to medical nutrition is to spoon feed the patient what they want to eat, if they are able to swallow. This is sometimes called **comfort feeding**. At the end of life, the patient's appetite declines and all they want is a few bites or a few sips of their favorite beverage. Their body cannot process food any longer, but this interaction of being fed is important for socialization and because of the meaning of eating.

Intuitively it seems clear that the National Cancer Institute (NCI) is right that with advanced directives, fewer patients with advanced cancer will undergo resuscitation and ventilator support and that these discussions need to begin early while patients are able to participate in decisions affecting their life.

A helpful statement of **decision-making capacity** was provided by the state of Florida, Department of Children and Families, in Tallahassee, on March 4, 2013. [198]

Decision-Making Capacity is judged to be.

(1) The capacity of a resident to:
(a) Understand his/her medical condition;
(b) Appreciate the consequences (benefits and burdens) of various treatment options including non-treatment;
(c) Judge the relationship between the treatment options and his/her personal values, preferences and goals;
(d) Reason and deliberate about his/her options; and,
(e) Communicate his/her decision in a meaningful manner.[199]

Writing about ventilator support the NCI report "The Last Days of Life," says

---

[198] Use of 'Do not Resuscitate' (DNR) Orders in State Mental Health Treatment Facilities. CF Operating procedure No. 155-52) (accessed Dec 28, 2013) (CFDP 155-52).
[199] CFDP 155-52, p. 2.

When ventilator support appears to be medically futile or is no longer consistent with the patient's (or family's or proxy's) goals of care, ventilator withdrawal to allow death may take place. Extensive discussions must first take place with patients (if they are able) and family members to help them understand the rationale for and process of withdrawal... Reframing the situation is helpful so that family members and significant others understand that the underlying disease process, and not ventilator withdrawal, is the cause of the patient's death.[200]

There is a helpful distinction between ordinary and extraordinary care. Ordinary care is familiar, accessible without unusual emotional or financial burden. Comfort feeding and even tube feeding would qualify as ordinary care in most instances. Extraordinary care is not the norm. The procedure may be new and carries emotional, financial or suffering burdens. Ventilator support would classify as extraordinary care and is thus not obligatory.

Comfort measures include pain medicine and medicines to help reduce a fever, oxygen, routine nursing care like keeping the patient clean and dry, emotional and spiritual support. "Any person who is in the end-stage of any disease process would be a candidate for a 'comfort care only' order and certainly for a hospice program."[201] Palliative care makes the distinction between killing and letting die; and distinctions between preserving life and preventing death. In comfort care, it would be prudent to add food and fluids, unless the patient is near death when the body cannot process these nutrients. Withholding food and fluids is closer to active killing than letting die. The most robust person can and will die without food and fluids. In the above section nutrition and hydration were included in ordinary care.

Patients in PVS are sometimes considered to have an end stage terminal illness. This is sometimes used as a reason to not feed these patients. They do not have the capacity to feed themselves and without food and fluids death occurs. Without medically prescribed food and fluids they would be dead. The argument goes something like this: in the pre-medical world they would have died, so let them die. The difficulty with this argument is that it can be used to not treat any disease condition one does not want to treat. Additionally, it does not seem reasonable to return to the pre-medical world.

Dunn writes "Many, if not most, hospice patients have been diagnosed with cancer. Yet more and more patients at home and in nursing homes

---

[200] "Last Days of Life"
http://www.cancer.gov/cancertopics/pdq/supportivecare/lasthours/healthprofession al (accessed December 31, 2013).
[201] Dunn, p.33.

suffering from dementia and other 'chronic' diseases are entering hospice care or having a 'comfort care only' treatment plan."[202] Comfort care provides support for the individual while not interrupting the natural course of the illness. This involves letting the patient die. This is a form of passive euthanasia providing for a peaceful death by not intervening. This seems true as long as comfort care includes food and fluids as desired by the patient. As we have seen, at the end of life when death is imminent the body cannot process food and fluids. The patient will only want a few bites and a few sips. At this point to provide tubal or intravenous fluids pushes fluid into the lungs and body tissues. Active euthanasia would be like assisted suicide, doing something to end the patient's life. Passive euthanasia fulfills moral expectations whereas active euthanasia generates many moral questions regarding conditions of informed consent and who has the right to end a life. It is not permitted in most states.

In comfort care the principle of double effect is emphasized. You will recall the principle of double effect says an action is permitted if (1) there is good intended as an end; (2) the means to achieve this end are not evil; (3) the undesirable side effect is only tolerated; and (4) there is a proportionally grave reason to tolerate the side effect. A common example is giving pain medication for the intention of comfort. With morphine there may be respiratory suppression making death a remote possibility, but the patient has been persistently suffering so the practitioner is willing to tolerate possible death. The death is not intended but tolerated. If the focus changes and death is our intention, then the principle of double effect no longer validates the action.

Conclusion

Capacities of health technology to extend life and prolong dying and the contemporary focus on autonomy have pushed the ill and their families into making difficult choices between life and death. We probably would not want it any other way, but this is a difficult choice leading to much ethical tension. "...before cardiopulmonary resuscitation was invented, when a patient stopped breathing, life was over."[203] In the end we will all die if the natural forces continue as they are. Twenty-five hundred years ago the first philosopher to study human life, Socrates, argued after being sentenced to death in the *Apology*, or defense of the philosophical life, that death is either nothingness resembling a deep sleep or a change of place to

---

[202] Dunn, p.34.
[203] Dunn, p.35.

the immaterial world. In either case, it is nothing to be feared if one has lived a good or virtuous life.[204]

There is a need to be precise with terminology and when practicing one especially needs to use the correct terminology. Is your patient brain dead? Is your patient in a coma or vegetative state? A coma patient will usually not have eyes open, but can transition to a vegetative state or conscious state. Patients in a vegetative state will have a sleep wake cycle and have opened eyes in wakefulness. "...there is a disassociation between wakefulness and awareness...there is a lack of evidence that the upper brain receives or projects information...the brain stem continues to manage the vegetative functions."[205] In contrast to the vegetative state, in a minimally conscious state or one experiencing focal brain injury or dementia, it is possible to suffer. Important in the diagnosis of a vegetative state is the lack of a "sustained and reproducible voluntary response." Fine adds, "Truly vegetative patients will not have reproducible responses to stimuli."[206]

Whether or not we have the "right-to-die" can be argued but we do have a right to refuse medical treatments even life-sustaining treatment based on a right to privacy (supported in the Quinlan case discussed earlier). In 1990 the US Supreme Court ruled in the case of Nancy Cruzan supporting that "patients have a fundamental right to refuse life-sustaining treatments but added that states may regulate the circumstances under which life sustaining treatments may be withdrawn when the patient cannot speak on his or her own behalf."[207]

One cannot do a little CPR but you can set a time limited trial.[208] Once CPR is begun you can see if your loved one will be one of those who respond successfully. If not you can take them off of the ventilator. The original event is killing them not removal of the ventilator. The ventilator just bought a little time to see if they would survive.

Cardiopulmonary resuscitation is not a required intervention. It is extraordinary care. It seems common in many ways because we are familiar with it, but it is extraordinary. Persons affirming administration for food and fluids or declining to remove the ventilator will sometimes assert they do not want to play God by letting them die. Then comes the response, but you are playing God in the prevention of death. And the rebuttal, if God wants them to die, they will die regardless of what is done.

---

[204] Fine, p.304.

[205] Plato, *Apology*, in the *Death and Trial of Socrates*, 3rd edition. Translated by G. M. A. Grube, Indianapolis: Hackett Publishing Company, 2000.

[206] Fine, p.304.

[207] Fine, p.305.

[208] Fine, p.306.

Conversation Starters:

a. What is it that provides a good and peaceful death for our loved ones and patients? Put yourself in the place of the dying. If you were dying, what would you see as required for a good and peaceful death.

b. It is natural to eat and natural to feed those who cannot feed themselves. It is considered natural to spoon feed, but isn't a spoon a delivery system like a feeding tube? Why is one considered natural and the other artificial?

c. If one of your loved ones was in a PVS and unable to feed themselves would you support or decline having them hand fed. Would you advice tube feeding?

d. If you were assigned to care for a patient from whom medical nutrition and hydration have been withdrawn? Would you be complicit in the person's death because you are caring for them? Support your answer.

e. What is your position and why do you hold that view (use ethical content), ought dementia patients to be treated with palliative or comfort care only? When an Alzheimer's dementia patient can no longer swallow, ought they to have a feeding tube inserted? Why or Why not?

Reflection Submissions:

1. To a great extent, decisions of whether or not to feed someone at the end of their life have been related to religious perspectives. Setting religious reasons aside, what leads to the requirement of providing food and fluid when the patient no longer feeds themselves? What argues we do not need to provide food and fluid in these same circumstances? Provide an argument from ethical principles for your personal position for or against providing food and fluids.

2. If clinical staff have rights of conscience, when caring for patients you have a right to practice health care in ways that preserve your values. What is your conscience position with end of life care? What do your values tell you to accept? What allows your participation?

Outline for Chapter 10: Issues at the End of Life
A. Parameters for Declaring Death
   1.Clinical death
   2. Brain death
   3. A case of brain death following cerebral anoxia
     a. Moral and ethical considerations of this case
     b. Confronting reality
     c. Personal moral decisions
     d. Health-care funding
     e. Practice concerns
   4. Brain death after severe head trauma
   5. When brain death does not occur
   6. The practitioner's role
     a. Judicial intervention
     b. A word of caution
B. Active and Passive Euthanasia
   1. Nutrition and hydration
     a. For organ donors
     b. Neurological deficits
   2. Enhancing life or preventing death
     a. Withholding foods and fluids
     b. Hard Choices for Loving People
     c. Mutual goal setting for supporting families
     d. Comfort care feeding
     e. The last days
   3. Resuscitation
     a. Values and concerns
C. Comfort Care and Letting Die
D. Conclusion

Terminology for Chapter 10
Clinical death
Brain death
Harvard criteria
Persistent or permanent vegetative state (PVS)
Coma
Active euthanasia
Passive euthanasia
Comfort feeding
Decision-making capacity

Chapter 11

Issues Related to Commitments, Professional Colleagues, Access to Health Care, and Institutions

Objectives

This chapter provides an opportunity for you to:

1. Describe actions of professional integrity within the student's discipline.
2. Describe the common-sense model of business ethics with applications to health care.
3. Describe the role of policies in allocation of scarce resources.
4. Define and compare rights and responsibilities.
5. List rights and responsibilities of a conscientious objector.
6. Describe government policies HIPPA, EEOC, Sexual Harassment.

Professionals are Human

By nature, humans are related to each other. Families celebrate birth and mourn death. As a class of being, we share the experience of having a human nature, which makes us both fragile and capable of excellence. Our pets participate in our communities as honorary humans. But humans are a different order or kind of being than animals because of our capacities for conceptual thought and freedom. We transcend ourselves in relationships and the care of others. This transcendence leads to development of formal and informal communities. At this level of involvement, we are members of families, groups, schools, churches, civic organizations.

The Law

We are citizens with natural and civil rights; natural rights secured by nature and civil rights being secured by human laws. As responsible citizens we participate in the development and governance of communities. From youth one must obey the laws and rules as the minimum expected to be a member of a community. It is said, the law is the minimum moral standard. You can at least obey the law. When we violate the law, we may be asked to show our willingness to change through fulfilling sanctions, or court assigned community service, or even incarceration. The violator is put in jail, not only as punishment and reformation, but also to protect the community. In a way this secures who can be trusted as a member of society and who cannot. These human laws are made by a legislative body for the peaceful running of society. Theoretically, they reflect moral standards the voting members of the community see as essential. There are many moral and virtuous expectations that are beyond requirements of the law. One's grasp of these standards and one's ability to fulfill them are determined by upbringing, religion, and education. It is about these moral issues that there are questions of discernment and application within specific circumstances.

Virtue

The inner force of human development pushes toward excellence or virtue. To review a bit, there are four cardinal virtues established in classical philosophy: (1) Prudence in knowing what is the case or what ought to be done; (2) Moderation or control of appetites and desires; (3) Courage that controls our contentious (angry) and fearful emotions; and (4) Justice or fairness in our interactions with self and others. Courage enables us to follow the wise decision, especially when we are afraid. (These virtues were developed in Chapter Six.)

As Professional

By education and licensure, we are related to communities of professionals. The bond among professionals of the same kind can be as close as, and closer than family. While civic communities are governed by political systems and legislative bodies who develop laws to be followed, professional communities are self-governed. The organizations have mission statements and codes of ethics that emerge from the beliefs and values of the profession.

An Example from a Professional Code

The professional code for Physical Therapists makes clear the relationship between values and ethical principles. After each core statement is a listing of values embraced by physical therapists, for example:

Principle #1: Physical therapists shall respect the inherent dignity and rights of all individuals. (Core Values: Compassion, Integrity);

Principle #2: Physical therapists shall be trustworthy and compassionate in addressing the rights and needs of patients/clients. (Core Values: Altruism, Compassion, Professional Duty).[209]

You may want to review the whole code as a trustworthy set of professional ethical statements and values. Since, a professional code can be a helpful guide, it is recommended that you locate and read your profession's code and make reference to it frequently. At every level of education and development you need to know your professional code.

Rules of Conduct

As a member of a community, civic or professional, you are expected to follow rules of conduct. As above, if one's behavior doesn't follow the rules of society, it indicates that you do not belong in the community. Professions govern themselves through entrance criteria and censure members who lapse in their performance of duties. This is usually the responsibility of the licensing board. Professional criteria include both content and conduct. The classic professionals are physicians, lawyers, and religious leaders. Today the term is expanded but still carries the meaning of striving for excellence in service or practice.

An Example of Rules of Conduct

The internet site for the Project Management Institute expresses well the role of all professions in guiding members and community expectations. If one does not abide by the established expectations one cannot be a member of the profession.

---

[209] http://www.apta.org/uploadedFiles/APTAorg/About_Us/Policies/HOD/Ethics/CodeofEthics.pdf (accessed January 19, 2015)

As practitioners of project management, *we are committed* to doing what is right and honorable. *We set high standards* for ourselves and we aspire to meet these standards in all aspects of our lives—*at work, at home, and in service to our profession.*

This Code of Ethics and Professional Conduct describes *the expectations* that we have of ourselves and our fellow practitioners in the global project management community. It articulates *the ideals* to which we aspire as well as *the behaviors that are mandatory* in our professional and volunteer roles.

The purpose of this Code is to instill confidence in the project management profession and to help an individual become a better practitioner. We do this by *establishing a profession-wide understanding of appropriate behavior.* We believe that the credibility and reputation of the project management profession is shaped by the collective conduct of individual practitioners.(Emphasis in italics added) [210]

The statement says all aspects of our lives, because the term "professional" characterizes a person and is not just about one's work-life. It is a way of being in community. This statement is very explicit and representative of the purpose of all codes to establish "a profession-wide understanding of appropriate behavior."

Integrity in Being and Doing

Professions are concerned with who you are as well as what you do. This requires integrity in being and doing. There are many persons working in health care who are not professionals, but the professional carries this extra social mandate in performance of their duties and in their personal conduct. To fulfill one's duties well does not require that one belong to a professional organization. Your membership is indicative of your commitment to your profession. For some areas of practice, there are certification examinations and professional state licensure. Scope or areas of practice are generally specified in this state licensure. Codes of ethics provide moral guidance but do not answer clinical practice questions.

Character and Integrity

What determines the morality of one's actions? How does this determination have application to life and work? Can you use the same standard for your private life and employment or professional life? These are important questions. It has been the insight of this book that both the

---

[210]   http://www.pmi.org/About- s/Ethics/~/media/PDF/Ethics/ap_pmicodeofethics .ashx (accessed January 7, 2014).

patient and the practitioner are human. Humanity forms a common bond and thus provides foundations for resolving ethical tensions in practice. Virtuous character and integrity assist in acting well. These foundations begin with training in youth and continue to develop as one respects standards of behavior throughout life. Virtue ethics express that what we do is who we are and who we become. So, we must act not only as we want to be treated (the ancient maxim) but in ways that develop who we want to be. Unique capacities found within being human lead one to act with respect for the value of human life and the dignity of each individual.

Michaud

My former colleague, Professor Thomas Michaud wrote of character and integrity in the lecture for chapter one in his book, *The Virtues of Business Ethics: Through Common Sense to Virtuous Common Decency.* Michaud really believed, and I agree, that a virtuous person with habits of good reasoning can discern the right thing to do in most situations.[211] He calls this virtuous common sense. The big gap is not in knowing what ought to be done, but in doing it.

Virtues Which Move to Action

The virtues of Prudence and Courage move a person from knowing the right action to doing it. Even more than a virtue, one needs a preponderance of virtue that might be called a virtuous character. We have already defined virtue as human excellence, a habit of acting well. Michaud teaches that a virtuous character is the primary source of ethical business practices.

Integrity

Michaud writes, "A person of integrity is not a divided self, a person who is in conflict with him or herself. A person of integrity is one whose personal moral values are integrated into his or her public work. Business people of integrity do not leave their moral values at home when they conduct business or do their work in a business."[212] The dominant insight in Michaud's work is that common sense can discern the moral if we strive to act with virtuous common decency, and when this becomes a habit we

---

[211] Acton, Massachusetts: Copley Custom Textbooks, pp. 24-28.

[212] Ibid, p.24.

are ethically empowered. We are able to "see" the right thing to do in a situation and do it. Assistance in finding the virtuous action is found in asking of the action: (1) is it legal (meets the law, codes and policies), (2) is it beneficial as a long term good for the community, and (3) is it honorable (would I be proud to be known as having done the action). Michaud calls this analysis the Common Sense Model of virtuous action.[213]

Health Care as a Business

It is no surprise that we have slipped into discussing business ethics. Health care is a business as much as it is human care. In terms of the beginning and end of life, ethical issues are deeply rooted in the meaning of life and preserving human dignity in health and illness, rehabilitation, and even death. In the intermediate, between the beginning and end of life, ethical questions revolve around how we ought to treat each other within complex situations. We are looking at successfully discerning the right thing to do and doing it in an interactive community system of health-care providers and patients/clients. Within the hospital or community health system, health-care providers and patients/clients are stable points in the complex of interpersonal interactions. (In the business of healthcare when the term client is used, the meaning includes patient.)

Legal

In a health-care setting, as within a corporation, the mission or vision ought to guide a statement of goals from which policies and rules are derived. Preceding the mission statement is a set of beliefs about life, health, business and the role of the health-care institution in the community and the country. Personal and corporate awareness of one's beliefs, mission and goals are significant in setting priorities and achieving desired outcomes. This flow is captured in the following chart.

Set of beliefs

Goals and then policies are made operational as rules and outcome criteria for evidence-based practice. Patients are self-determining humans who require knowledge of their health condition, past interventions, and potential outcomes in order to participate in their health- care decisions.

---

[213] Ibid, p.8.

Better outcomes result from mutually set goals as health practitioners and patients work together to achieve desired health ends.[214] Within the complexity of the health-care setting one can also identify the rights and responsibilities framed by employment contracts. Part of consideration of what is a legal action is an understanding of rights (what you are entitled to as human and as participating in your contract as an employee and as a professional) and responsibilities (duties related to being human, holding a particular position and participating as a professional). The minimal ethical standard for health-care professionals is "doing no harm" (non-malfeasance).

Mission or Vision statement
↓
Goals
↓
Policies
↓
Rules
↓
Outcome criteria

Chart 2: Flow Chart from Beliefs to Outcomes

Beneficial

Being a benefit to yourself, your family, your patients/clients, institution or company, community and country moves one beyond doing no harm to doing the beneficial. Beneficence[215] is actually hard to achieve. Many actions may benefit yourself and/or your family, or patient, but not the health-care institution or community at large. Often what appears to benefit only one's self or one's family, patients/clients, or department is only a short-term benefit that does not characterize the action as the best that can be done in the situation. Decisions of beneficence, or long-term benefit, usually require identification of stakeholders and analysis of both short and long term benefits of each stakeholder. One has to be able to imaginatively project short and long-term outcomes. One must also decide what counts as a benefit. Some believe the needs and fair or just treatment of individuals must be evaluated against the needs of the institution or

---

[214] The importance of mutually set goals is discussed and developed by Imogene King, *Theory for Nursing, Systems, Concepts, Process.* Wiley and Sons,1981.
[215] Beneficence is also part of Principlism which was previously discussed

company or community and fair (just) treatment of all stakeholders. This consideration of outcomes is often called a "**cost/benefit analysis**."[216]

Honorable

Doing the honorable means being proud of an action. One can ask, would I want my wife, family, patients, community, supervisor, professional colleagues, or CEO to know I chose this action. If you can live with yourself, that's minimal, but this standard, the honorable, calls you to act with a pride and integrity that promotes the good of your community.

Allocation of Scarce Resources[217]

Within health care practice, allocation decisions are especially poignant because the well-being and lives of individuals are at risk. In health care ethics, we say, every life is valuable and every individual deserving of care. However, when there is no money or when there are not enough supplies to go around, this position does not mean that resources can or ought to be dispersed to meet the needs of all persons. The ethical tension generated by these realities (persons in need and insufficient supplies) is moderated when one believes that he or she has made the best decision possible within the difficult presenting circumstances. This kind of a decision seems beyond the analysis provided by the legal, the beneficial, and the honorable. Yet, they provide some distinct assistance and we would be benefited by taking these ideas into consideration.

Legal

One must discriminate, to discern between persons according to those whose condition can and cannot likely be improved. It seems the legal requirement of equal treatment cannot be met, and yet there can be no

---

[216] See R. M. Veatch, *The Basics of Bioethics, 2nd edition.* Upper Saddle River: Prentice Hall, p.121-139.

[217] This work is largely from lectures and university e-articles that were written. "Allocation of scarce resources: wisdom from contemporary management and classical philosophy," *eCardinal Perspectives* 2008-9. And, "Ethical Decision-making with Distribution of Scarce Resources," *eCardinal Perspectives* 2004-5. "Allocation of Scarce Resources: wisdom from contemporary management and classical philosophy," at the conference "Nursing Ethics and Health Care Policy; Bridging Local, National and International Perspectives" International Center for Nursing Ethics. Yale University, New Haven, CT, July 18, 2008.

discrimination according to race, gender, sexual orientation, national origin and culture. The critical discernment is between likelihood of benefit or no benefit from treatment based on the health condition of the individual and what resources it would take to provide needed care. If we were emergency responders, we would be protected from being sued by the persons assisted and their families according to the Good Samaritan Laws. One must still practice within usual and expected standards of practice.

Beneficial

Long term benefit would ask care providers to be transparent so the community would continue to trust them.

Honorable

If this is an emergency, a major crisis, calling for triage and a determination of who will be cared for, questions of honor seem irrelevant. Yet, at the "end of the day" when all is said and done, one needs to feel "I served well;" that "I did my best."

As clinical practitioners you may be expected to implement community or institutional allocation plans. In some instances, you may be asked to participate as an emergency management committee member. As a valued member of this team you will discuss and assist the committee in setting policies that balance the needs of individual people and organizations against available resources and the needs of the whole community (or country).

Justice in the distribution of goods and services asks if society's benefits and burdens ought to be divided equally among all citizens, or according to contribution, or need. Aristotle would argue for **equity**, distribution according to actual or potential contribution. Christian doctrine argues for care of the poor and weak, leading many to assert distribution according to need. Political doctrine also divides on this matter: conservatives arguing that care of those in need ought to be through voluntary contributions and community non-governmental agencies; liberals arguing that the role of government is to care for citizens.

Fair Distribution Requires Balance

The first thing organizations need to do in times of scarcity is to use resources more efficiently. But when after more efficient use of what is available, there is still insufficient funding, personnel and supplies to meet the needs of all, the challenge is, how does one fairly distribute what is available? This includes who will receive services, as well as getting the greatest benefit out of money, personnel and supplies. Justice requires that the system of delivery balance human need and human dignity with effective outcomes in the use of resources or possible treatment options depending on the situation one is facing. Imagine a balance with three measuring pans. You have seen the classic Scales of Justice with two pans for weighing the crime and punishment. This allocation balance has three pans. With allocation decisions there are three things to be held in balance: (1) needs of individuals and groups; (2) available resources; and (3) valued outcomes. Needs of individuals must be measured against available resources and resources must be used where they can maximize positive results. No one knows the future. Outcomes must be projected by people knowledgeable from past experience and an understanding of risks and benefits. This kind of determination requires knowledge of the situation (the injuries or health needs of patients), the capacities of available personnel, and supplies available, and projected outcomes. This determination is the role of triage leadership. There are no easy answers. The best results follow guidelines and decisions made from experience. The leader needs knowledge and a stable character of justice and concern. To prevent bias or conflict of interest, this triage leader ought not to be the clinician serving patients within those needing the scarce supplies.

Policies are Gatekeepers

Policies are extremely important gatekeepers for fair distribution. They depersonalize acceptance and rejection of individual patients and set standards for clinicians and agency personnel. Policies stand between general philosophical principles of ethical practice, like valuing life and justice, and specific allocation decisions. Ideally, if the policies are well developed the decision becomes whether or not the individual or the situation fits within the policy, thus, reducing a potentially complex ethical decision into one of clinical or organizational management; the person qualifies or they do not. Clearly stated, (1) allocation of scarce resources requires careful use of personnel and supplies available, and (2) evaluation of the patient/client receiving the services ought to be based on needs, potential to recover, and capacity of the patient/client to effectively use the resources. This assessment will facilitate getting the greatest benefit out of health care dollars spent. Distributive justice requires that the system of care delivery balance human need and human dignity with effectiveness of outcomes of possible placement or treatment options to avoid harm and maximize quality of life.

In his book about tiny newborns, *Too Expensive to Treat: Finitude, Tragedy and Neonatal ICU*, Charles Camosy[218] also frames this essential dichotomy between the clinical perspective where there are no limits to what ought to be done and the finitude of resources. We accept that every life is precious, but there is also the business side of health care where there must be limits. Budgets must be kept; bills and salaries must be paid. Policies are made in the abstract, but care is given to particular individuals. Given these dynamics, tension and controversy are inevitable; perhaps even necessary, to achieve a middle ground.

Rights and Responsibilities

Rights divide into natural rights and civil rights, as previously noted. Rights are actions and things to which we are entitled (positive rights) or to non-interference (negative rights) as in our search for happiness.

Natural Rights

These rights are secured by the kind of being we are as human, with capacities for knowledge and choice. Expressed by the United States Declaration of Independence, they are the inalienable right to life, liberty, and the pursuit of happiness. These are our negative rights, our right to non-interference in our person. You are not allowed to take my life or my freedom. The irony is that the founders of our country, the writers of the Declaration, many if not most, were slave owners. These words of the Declaration first penned in 1776 have taken 200 years to become reality.

Civil Rights

These rights are secured by law, the legal norms of a community or country. The Emancipation Proclamation of Abraham Lincoln was in 1863, and the Civil Rights Movement was in the 1950's and 60's. "The Civil Rights Act of 1964 prohibits discrimination of all kinds based on race, color, religion, or national origin." This law even provided for forced desegregation.[219] Interestingly, in 1964 the Civil Rights Act was only for

---

[218] Grand Rapids, Michigan: William B. Eerdmans Publishing Company, 2010.

[219] http://www.infoplease.com/spot/civilrightstimeline1.html (accessed January 15, 2014).

equality among men. We note that the Equal Rights Amendment securing equality for women passed in the U.S. Senate and House of Representatives in 1972 but was only ratified by 35 states so did not change the Constitution. Additionally, the 14th amendment (ratified 1868) secured all privileges and protections under the law for all men, but the 19th amendment (ratified 1920) secured only voting rights for women, not equal protections.[220] Protections for children, and child welfare rights came from organizations for protection of animals in the 1960's. Although taking a long time, 200 years later, we are seeing the fulfillment of the Declaration of Independence well beyond the vision of our founding fathers. Current interpretation of the Declaration itself, can be seen to include men, women and children.

Where negative rights secure freedom from interference, positive rights are entitlements, like government supported education. Democratic participative government requires informed citizens to vote, so we have government sponsored education. Because we have a natural right to life, it could be argued we have a right to food and shelter, as well as the right to not be attacked and killed. On the basis of this inalienable right to life, there are laws against suicide. Police can detain a homeless person to sleep in a shelter when the temperature is life-threateningly hot or cold. This natural right to life also seems to argue for access to health care for all persons.

Rights and Responsibilities are Reciprocal

For every right there is at least one responsibility. If you have a right to life, you have a responsibility to preserve yourself. In the preceding section we discussed a right to be exempt from participation in an action against your conscience beliefs. To claim this right, you have a responsibility to make your position known and be willing to accept a different assignment. If you have a right to health care, you have a responsibility to fulfill prescriptions and follow advice that will preserve or restore your health. There is also a responsibility to pay for these services. The one responsible for providing health services has a right to be paid, to have the cost of services compensated fairly. The question becomes who is responsible to pay for services when the patient cannot.

There was a wonderful hospital in downtown Washington, D.C. It primarily served very poor and homeless patients. The social services staff would file for Medicaid and where possible, Medicare, but there was just not enough reimbursement to keep the hospital open. It was a sad day

---

[220] http://womenshistory.about.com/od/equalrightsamendment/a/equal_rights_
amendment_overview.htm (accessed January 15, 2014).

when the hospital closed its doors and many poor and homeless living in that area were no longer able to receive care. Free clinics in the area filled in for services as they were able. Hospitals depend on sufficient insured or private paying patients to pay both their expenses and the expenses of those without insurance or insufficient insurance. Whether insured or not, one expects to receive health care if needed. There is a requirement that a person must be stabilized in the Emergency Room, but the hospital does not have to admit the patient if uninsured. Many communities have clinics for those unable to pay for care, and some hospitals do have plans for charity care but even non-profit organizations must have a balanced budget or they close.

As an employee you have the right to a safe working environment and the equipment to fulfill your professional responsibilities. Reciprocally you have the responsibility for the judicious use of equipment and supplies, not taking supplies for personal use, and being careful to record charges. There is also an obligation to your employer for the proper use of your time and care of durable equipment. Concurrently, the employer has a responsibility to provide needed equipment and the right to expect professional practice.

Conscientious Objections

Accommodations for a conscientious objection based on religious beliefs are generally protected. Conscientious objectors must notify their supervisor as soon as possible if it is expected the objectionable event may occur. As one example, pro-life practitioners on rotation may be serving in an operating room when it becomes expected they will assist a woman having an abortion. When an objection occurs, there is a need to change assignments and cover for the objector's absence. If you are the objector, you have the right to accommodation, but you must request it responsibly and respectfully. Without a prior plan, information must be obtained, administration must be notified and a decision has to be made quickly. It will be much easier for faculty and supervisors to support your non-participation if you have expressed objections from the beginning or at least long before the event. Accommodation as a conscientious objector requires a consistent and stable background that supports the objection of practicing in these situations. It is unacceptable that one decides and requests accommodation on the day they are called to act.

Government Regulations

Health Insurance Portability and Accountability Act of 1996 (HIPAA)

Anyone working in health care today needs to be familiar with the Health Insurance Portability and Accountability Act of 1996 (HIPAA). These are Privacy Rules that secure an individual's health information but allows disclosure to insurance companies for evaluation and payment to health-care providers. You will notice the HIPPA statement reads, "…the Privacy Rule is balanced so that it permits the disclosure of health information needed for patient care and other important purposes."[221] Every health-care office and department has patients sign privacy disclosure forms and has policies against unlawful disclosure that could result in the loss of one's job. In the private disclosure of information there is no longer a moral question, it is illegal. The ethical discussion is or not to report violations.

Understanding Health Information Privacy

The HIPAA Privacy Rule provides federal protections for individually identifiable health information held by covered entities and their business associates and gives patients an array of rights with respect to that information. At the same time, the Privacy Rule is said to be balanced as it permits the disclosure of health information needed for patient care and other important purposes.

The Security Rule specifies a series of administrative, physical, and technical safeguards for covered entities and their business associates to use to assure the confidentiality, integrity, and availability of electronic protected health information.[222]

Equal Employment Opportunity Commission (EEOC)

No statement of rights would be complete without treatment of EEOC[223] that secures equal employment opportunities. You will note that

---

[221] http://www.hhs.gov/ocr/privacy/hipaa/understanding/index.html (accessed, January 15, 2014)

[222] From handout by Perry Bryant, WVAHC, April 19, 2012 (West Virginians for Affordable Health Care). For further information (http://www.warresisters.org/node/328) (accessed January 16, 2014).

[223] http://www.eeoc.gov (accessed January 15, 2014).

this equal rights act of 1964 was amended to include sexual discrimination. For the most part, being treated respectfully in the work place is now a matter of law. There are still issues that emerge with employers not enforcing the requirements or not hearing what the person is saying when they are filing a complaint.

Your Rights[224]

Private Employment, State and Local Governments, Educational Institutions

Applicants to and employees of most private employers, state and local governments, educational institutions, employment agencies and labor organizations are protected under the following Federal laws:

Race, Color, Religion. Sex. and National Origin

Title VII of the Civil Rights Act of 1964, as amended, prohibits discrimination in hiring, promotion, discharge, pay, fringe benefits, job training, classification, referral, and other aspects of employment, on the basis of race, color, religion, sex or national origin.

Disability

The Americans with Disabilities Act of 1990, as amended, protects qualified applicants and employees with disabilities from discrimination in hiring, promotion, discharge, pay, job training, fringe benefits, classification, referral, and other aspects of employment on the basis of disability. The law also requires that covered entities provide qualified applicants and employees with disabilities with reasonable accommodations that do not impose undue hardship.

Age Discrimination

The Age Discrimination in Employment Act of 1967, as amended, protects applicants and employees 40 years of age or older from discrimination on the basis of age in hiring, promotion, discharge, compensation, terms, conditions or privileges of employment.

Sex Discrimination

In addition to sex discrimination prohibited by Title VII of the Civil Rights Act of 1964, as amended (see above), the Equal Pay Act of 1963, as amended, prohibits sex discrimination in payment of wages to women and men performing substantially equal work in the same establishment.

---

[224] http://www.ushistory.org/Declaration/document/ (assessed January 15, 2014).

Retaliation against a person who files a charge of discrimination, participates in an investigation, or opposes an unlawful employment practice is prohibited by all of these Federal laws. If you believe that you have been discriminated against under any of the above laws, you should immediately contact an attorney to determine your rights.

Sexual Harassment

Protection from unwanted sexual verbal and physical contact is guaranteed under the EEOC guidelines. Your refusal to participate or your complaint about advances, cannot legally lead to your loss of employment. This is part of your security of person. You have a right to safety and to do your work in peace. Harassment may be an expectation of favors to secure your position, or the unpleasant impact on the work environment of nude pictures, lewd jokes, or undesired touching. Notice to be harassment the behavior has to be undesired. It may still be inappropriate, but if you are not offended or do not express that you are offended, it is not harassment. Reportable sexual harassment either quid pro quo (to secure a position) or hostile environment (to heckle or tease) requires repeated offenses with requests that the behavior stop. Sometimes hostile work environment or sexual harassment charges stem from a difference in culture. In some areas it is common to say "hon," "dearie," or "sugar." Someone from another part of the country might say, "How can you let him (or her) talk to you like that." "What! He doesn't mean anything by it." "I sure wouldn't put up with it." To one it is acceptable, the other not. Harassment is very individually defined, but if one were doing or saying something and was asked to stop, he or she ought to do so to avoid charges. Early in my career teaching Philosophy, I had a very difficult experience. I was teaching in the evening and every evening an older male professor would come into the classroom, take out the overhead projector and stop to 'tease' a lovely young lady in my class. I was very upset and spoke to the neutral third party representative on campus. She said it had to be offensive to the student. It was not. The student said she had been a bartender and was used to guys talking like that. Anyway, she said she had been in his class before, so she knew he meant no harm. So, I was the one offended and I had to speak with the professor. I did. He said he was embarrassed that he had to come into my class every night to get the equipment he needed to teach his class. He had asked that the equipment be available but it never was. Whether I believed his reason or not I had a solution. Every evening I moved the equipment into the hall. In this process, I surely had to be courageous, probably the most important of all the virtues. I also, had to decide if I would be humble and move the equipment or insist he stop being the flirt in my class. Sometimes there is wisdom in finding a middle ground, avoiding the confrontation. Actually, being humble was easier than confronting a full professor my having just started a new job.

Conclusion: Everyday Ethics

As described earlier in this chapter, health institutions are founded on statements of beliefs about patients, health and healing expressed as mission statements. These mission or vision statements are the foundation of policies and expectations made of employees. Policies and employment practices are important for the smooth running of an organization. Employees are expected to be aware of these policies and employment practices.

This text has connected Philosophy and philosophical inquiry to health-care practices. Philosophy asks the big conceptual questions: being human, environment, the meaning of health and illness, being a practitioner and being a patient. Every clinical action is particular; an exchange between this client and this caregiver. Philosophical perspectives are broad universal statements. Philosophy asks us to be aware of our beliefs, values and prejudices because they guide interpretation of situations and guide decision making.

Individuals are called to be moral. This morality must guide how we act every day to be a viable part of our lives. Whether with family, friends, patients or professional colleagues all people are to be treated with respect. The reason for this is the kind of beings we are in our involvement in interactions, whether on the simplest or most stressful day. Additionally, as human our character is made by what we do. By acting with patience, we are more and more patient. When we act rudely, we become rude. When we act, we are more likely to repeat the action done. We form virtuous habits by acting with virtue. Humans are also the beings capable of knowledge and choice. Humans deserve to be respected and to have their decisions respected if they are made with intent and capacity. We do these things every day. We collaborate with friends and family. We do not expect to walk into a room and tell everyone what to do.

On the average day, we are called to treat patients as valued individuals. They need to be treated with respect, just as our family does. We elicit their permission to touch them, to do the required test or treatment. We keep our word, and work in ways that promote their well-being. In professional practice one's professional capacities are added to the ordinary ethical treatment of people. Every day we are called to treat people well, that is, to be moral. Occasionally, we encounter the difficult decisions; then we utilize the principles and ideas of Ethics, but every day we are called to act with informed ordinary, common courtesy. Every day we confront allocation of scarce resources in the use of our time when deciding what to do whether for our family and friends or when working as a practitioner.

Conversation Starters:

1. For the following situations, summarize your analysis for each of these considerations of the Common Sense Model, as well as your decision of what ought to be done. (Benefit has been added for clarity.)

   What is legal (includes policies and codes)?

   What is of benefit (short term good)?

   What provides beneficence (long term good)?

   What is honorable?

   Use these questions to clarify what needs to be done, and why?

   a. As you walk into the nurse's station to page your colleague for assistance, you see the unit secretary quickly close an eBay site. He nervously says he was just checking to see if his bid was accepted.

   b. In what significant ways do your reflections and responses change if this is a frequent occurrence?

   c. As you enter the medical records library, two hospital employees are looking through a chart and laughing (snickering) and pointing at items on the pages.

   d. Your colleague, Pat, comes to work 15-20 minutes late 2-3 times a week. The excuse is the school bus driver is late. You now know this is not true as a friend's children began riding the same bus. Do you think you need to question accuracy of shift records prepared by Pat? This pattern of being late emerged slowly and you have just been covering the workload. Now that you know Pat is not providing the real reason for being late, you no longer want to cover the work. Use the above analysis and the following options to decide what ought you to be done?

   (1) Continue to cover for Pat even though you do not want to in the hope to one day receive a favor in return.

   (2) Ask for an explanation and threaten to go to the supervisor if you do not like the explanation. (3) Ask the supervisor to implement a time card system.

   (4) Tell Pat you can no longer pretend nothing is wrong and call the supervisor when Pat does not arrive on time.

   (5) Other. Provide a principle-based reason for your answer.

2. You are on the admissions board of a prominent university. A 19-year-old with conviction of burglary and theft at age 16 is applying for admission as a prelaw student. You have had the experience of admitting a student with a police record before. They completed at the university, even law school, then were not allowed to sit for the

Bar exam. Reportedly, there was a question if they met the character requirements. Provide answers and principle-based reasons for your decisions.

   a. Ought professions be allowed to restrict someone capable of the academic work?

   b. Would you recommend the person for regular admission or provisional admission to the university?

   c. Does the admissions committee have a responsibility to question this admission?

3. Your colleague arrives to replace you having the faint smell of alcohol. What action would you take?

   Provide answers and principle-based reasons for your decisions in the following circumstances:

   a. You are expected home in 15 minutes to care for your son so your spouse can go to work.

   b. You are expected home to take your 2 year old son to the doctor because he has a high fever?

4. Hospitals routinely charge for items the patients did not use, say, protective pads for the bed. A call to billing about this would reveal that everyone has these charges to make up for supplies for which they cannot charge. Would you assess this to be moral? Whether you hold this practice is moral or not, suggest alternatives. Support your position.

Reflection Submissions:

1. Provide arguments to show health-care is a right, or that it is not a right but a human need that people ought to fulfill for themselves? Support your answer.

2. Provide your arguments (with supporting premises), does charitable care of the poor through private agencies promote human dignity and freedom, or are citizens better served by distribution of funds according to need from centralized monies collected as taxes (government)?

3. Where is the highest priority between each paired option? Support your position. Can you suggest a middle ground? Support your suggested middle ground option.

   (a) Within an emergency, ought there to be care of all individuals in immediate need **or** holding on to some supplies, not dispensing them at this time in case something worse happens?

   (b) First care for local residents then consider strangers because we have a greater responsibility to our own **or** assess and distribute

supplies just based on need and potential for recovery?
    (c) Requiring legal residency papers to receive care **or** assess and distribute just based on need and potential for recovery.
4. Tiny newborns, under 500 grams (16 ounces), usually suffer physical and mental defects if they survive early infancy. Ought taxpayer dollars to be spent trying to save these littlest human babies? Answer for the clinician working with the family and child; and then for those legislating state policies for allocation of scarce resources. Be sure to support your position with moral/ethical principles.
5. One of my favorite memories while visiting in the nursing home was seeing two elderly ladies walking hand in hand, pushing an imaginary grocery cart. You could hear them speaking and giggling but it was not possible to know what they were saying. It looked as if they were talking about what they were buying as they picked desired items from the imaginary groceries they saw on the wall.

   In an economy with a very tight health-care budget, is it right to spend public funds keeping alive those who only have imaginary experiences? Provide your reasoning that they should or should not be cared for.

   If one says those with dementia ought not to be preserved with public funds, what about the profoundly retarded or mentally ill? Where would you draw the line? Be sure to support your position with moral/ethical principles.

Outline for Chapter 11: Issues Related to Commitments, Professional Colleagues, Access to Health Care and Institutions
    A. The Professionals as Humans
        1. The law
        2. Virtue
        3. As professional
            a. An example from a professional code
            b. Code of Conduct
            c. An example of rules of contact
        4. Integrity in Being and Doing
    B. Character and Integrity
        1. Michaud
        2. Virtues which move to action
        3. Integrity

C. Heath Care as a Business
1. Legal
2. Beneficial
3. Honorable
D. Allocation of Scare Resources
1. Legal
2. Beneficial
3. Honorable
4.Fair distribution requires balance
D. Policies and Gatekeepers
E. Rights and Responsibilities
1. Natural rights
2. Civil rights
3. Rights and responsibilities are reciprocal
F. Conscientious Objections
G. Government Regulations
1. Health Insurance Portability and Accountability Act of 1196 (HIPAA)
2. Understanding health information privacy
3. .Equal Employment Opportunity commission (EEOC)
4. Your Rights
   a. Race, color, religion, sex, and national origin
   b. Disability
   c. Age discrimination
   d. Sex discrimination
5.Sexual harassment
H. Conclusion: Everyday Ethics

Terminology for Chapter 11
Cost/benefit analysis
Equity
Integrity
Natural rights
Civil rights

APPENDICES:
TEACHER'S GUIDE

The purpose of this teacher's guide is to provide support for the planning and teaching of lessons from *Humanity at the Heart of Practice: Philosophical Ethics for Health Care*. The outcome expectations for courses which use this textbook are for students to (1) make decisions in moral situations by the application of principles of philosophical ethics, (2) understand the foundations of the philosophical principles compatible with the students own personal informal moral development, and (3) to resolve ethical dilemmas into their essential components using a provided framework to make clear the conflicting values, policies, or principles. This analysis of ethical situations will allow the student to reason to a principle-based solution. In the interactive classroom, students will be able to explore alternative views and gain an awareness of self, culture, and contemporary moral issues. It is believed students who take this course will gain some of the capacities and insights usually provided by a humanities curriculum.

The teacher's guide will provide: chapter-by-chapter overviews, chapter outlines and new terminology teaching strategies, classroom activities, and commentary on select conversation starters and reflection submissions. It is our hope these tools will assist teachers to combine the information provided into plans for each chapter that will facilitate learning within the teacher's context.

APPENDIX A:
CHAPTER OVERVIEWS

This appendix provides insights about philosophical ethics and the organizing structure of the book. The discipline of Ethics is the study of proper human action, what ought to be done to further the human good. This 'ought' is related to living a happy or excellent human life; one characterized by virtue and could be said to be virtuous. A virtue is a habit of acting well. One of the earliest philosophers and the first to write an ethics text was Aristotle (4th Century. BC). He taught that one could not study Ethics without having virtue, because without virtue you would not recognize moral principles which are the starting points for analyzing and deciding within situations having moral tensions. The scope of philosophical ethics includes the meaning of human life, the human good, human excellence, a just society, individual and corporate virtue, principles of practice, and the process of ethical-decision making. Theological ethics begins with acceptance of a Supreme Being and uses teachings within what are believed to be revealed documents. These are outside the scope and practice of Philosophy. It is often said that Philosophy is concerned with what can be known in the light of human reason, thus it is concerned with knowledge of our world and good argumentation. And yet, these are not enough to explain human action. People are moved to action by what they value, not just what they know. Philosophers use teachings from revealed content if they can reason logically to see how the theological content fits with the inquiry.

Our society generally, and health care in particular, are brimming with questions. Is it really better for people to make their own treatment decisions? Wasn't it easier, simpler and less worrisome when the doctor just told you what treatment you needed? Is the average person able to quickly grasp enough information to make an informed decision, the doctor has gone to school for several years to know what ought to be done? On the other hand, what right does anyone have to tell another person what to do? It is their life. Some people assert, if what I do doesn't affect anyone else, I can do whatever I want. The philosophy asks, "Is it possible that an individual can act and no one else be effected?"

Actually, if all persons are related, then there is something that unites humans in America, Africa, China, Europe and the Middle East. Humans are the beings in the world who are concerned with what ought to be done, and they receive the impact of another human's action good or evil, moral or immoral, so this book uses humanity, relationships, and ethical decision-making as its organizing core content. The early pages provide important content about values, ideas, terms and logic helpful for understanding the rest of the book.

Section One: Values and Practical Reasoning

Chapter 1: Values

An inquiry into your own values and the role of values in one's life begins your experience of thinking philosophically. Proper human conduct, i.e. moral action begins with childhood training in virtue. These virtuous habits of acting well lead to excellent, peaceful living. The reality that the professional practitioner is first a human, born within a culture and having good days and bad days, sets the foundation for development of professional ethics.

Chapter 2: Practical Reasoning

This chapter is a consideration of philosophical inquiry, concepts and reasoning. Students are introduced to the practical syllogism and its role in clinical practice and moral decisions. There also is an introduction of normative principles that provide moral guidance and the idea that there are principles of ethical practice within humanity itself.

Section Two: Philosophical Perspectives of Nature and Human Nature

Chapter 3: Foundations of Knowing Nature and Human Nature

Classical philosophy guides our understanding of the world, providing principles of stability and change. It is interesting that what is known comes to be known through the principle of stability, the form, which makes us be the kind of existent being that we are, human, dog or flower. Nevertheless, what we experience in the world are particular matter/form individuals, Jeff, Rover or a rose. After a short introduction to formal logic this chapter provides an Aristotelian explanation of nature, human nature and acquiring knowledge.

Chapter 4: Humans as Persons in Community

Extending the thinking of nature to human nature leads one to awareness of the immateriality of the intellect. This immateriality places humanity as a unique kind of being in the world. There is consideration of essential human attributes and their emergence, as well as origins of human dignity. Experiences of practitioners in the early days of advanced technology challenge the meaning of care. Norris Clarke adds to our understanding of being human with the awareness that we are persons in community. This chapter concludes with the work of the Nurse Educator Imogene King. It is believed that clinical theory bridges philosophy and practice.

Section Three: Persons

Chapter 5: The Practitioner is First a Human Then a Professional

The practitioner is first a human with strengths and weaknesses who must first care for themselves and then for others. While there are many kinds of caring, healing practice requires a culture of integrity. Professionals have a mandate from society with government licensure. Science provides a stable base of organized knowledge generated by documented controlled inquiry. This is the science of practice. The art of clinical practice is the skillful, experienced application of disciplinary knowledge within particular situations.

Chapter 6: The Patient is Also a Person

The intent of this chapter is to see the vulnerable presenting person as more than a patient or client for the practice of my specialty or yours. Education and knowledge from practice give the professional a responsibility to intervene, if possible, to ease the distress of persons in their care. This chapter considers situations of vulnerability and the moral responsibility that comes with recognizing this vulnerability. Also considered are principles which emerge from the lawfulness of the universe that are the basis of Natural Law Ethics.

Section Four: Ethical reasoning and Ethical Theories

Chapter 7: The Right Action Requires Discernment and Virtue

Discernment requires knowledge of the situation one is confronting, knowledge of one's view of the human good, codes, policies, law and of ethical principles. In addition to all of these aspects of knowing, doing the right action also requires virtue, practical wisdom for knowing what ought to be done, and the courage for doing it. As a discipline, ethics doesn't usually tell people what they have to do in specific situations. In a similar way philosophy highlights, organizes, clarifies, and recommends. Philosophy provides insight into the decision-making process. It provides new ways of thinking about things or events and helps to answer questions. This chapter provides an overview of ethical decision-making and a tool for analysis of dilemmas.

Chapter 8: A Short Overview of Philosophical Ethical Perspectives

Philosophers today ask the same kinds of questions that have been asked for thousands of years. Technology and scientific progress confront a thoughtful person with new dilemmas for the application of principles but principles have not changed. For this reason, we consider the writings of the wise people who have gone before. This text provides answers most often from the works of Plato and Aristotle, but there are important insights from other philosophers that will also assist students within their clinical practice. It is believed in studying ethics one gains in virtue, which increases the capacity to resolve moral dilemmas and to live an excellent human life. It is believed ethical insight into the situated human good is facilitated by an understanding of nature, humanity and the place of humans in the world.

Section Five: Humanity at the Heart of Practice

Chapter 9: Ethical Issues Related to the Beginning of Life

This chapter will specifically consider the difficult question of when human life begins. Because practitioners work within a hospital system it is necessary to begin with questions of accountability and implied consent. Scientific and philosophic content will allow one to argue for and against positions related to select issues confronted at the beginning of life, abortion, IVF and embryonic stem cell research.

Chapter 10: Issues at the End of Life

Ethical decisions at the end of life require distinctions between anoxic brain injury and traumatic brain death. It is also important to consider when a person is dead; interventions that prevent death but do not promote life, substituted judgment and health care agency. This chapter will confront interventions that are natural and artificial, ordinary and extraordinary, and the important distinctions between killing and letting die, and palliative versus futile care.

Chapter 11 Issues Related to Commitments, Professional Colleagues, Access to Health Care and Institutions

This chapter is concerned with professional practice and issues that arise with health care as a business in a world of scarce resources, including the practitioner's time, finances within the health-care system, and items like transplantable organs. It is concerned with preservation of integrity and fulfilling one's responsibilities to policies and regulations, including governmental policies of HIPPA, EEOC, and prevention of sexual harassment.

APPENDIX B:
CHAPTER OUTLINES AND NEW TERMINOLOGY

Section One: Values

Outline for Chapter 1: Values

A. Introduction
B. Ethical Decisions are Similar to Clinical Decisions
C. Community Values
D. Personal Values
    1. Ethical dilemmas
    2. Management decisions
    3. Common moral decisions
E. Seeking the Principle-based Action
    1. Equality is a principle
Terminology for Chapter 1
Moral or ethical tensions
Dilemmas

Outline for Chapter 2: Practical Reasoning

A. Introduction to Arguments
B. Coming to Know Concepts
    1. Mathematical concepts
    2. Non-mathematical concepts
    3. Concepts build arguments
C. Two Ancient Laws of Thought
    1. The principle of identity
    2. The principle of non-contradiction
D. Being Philosophical
    1. Metaphysic as a division of philosophy
    2. The philosophy of nature
    3. Mathematics used by philosophers
    4. Ethics is a study of proper human action
    5. The logic of practical reasoning

E. Study of Informal Logic
   1. An example of deductive practical reasoning
   2. An example of inductive practical reasoning
   3. Arguments secure decisions not actions
   4. A question of justice as an example of ethical reasoning
   5. Two levels of logical discussion
F. Philosophical Answers and Normative Principles
   1. Normative principles
   2. Principles within humanity
   3. Human dignity
   4. Inherent human dignity
   5. Socially attributed dignity
G. Conclusion

Terminology for Chapter 2
Argument
Propositions
Premises
Conclusion
Inductive argument
Deductive argument
Concepts
Universals
Conclusion
Premises
Tautology
Univocal
Equivocal
Equivocation
Philosophical
Metaphysics
Natural philosophy
Ethics
Practical reasoning
Moral maxim
Claims
Inductive
Deductive
Valid argument
Sound argument
Practical wisdom
Practical syllogism

Normative
Relativism
Nonmaleficence
Justice
Autonomy
Beneficence
Principlism
Dignity
Inherent dignity
Attributed dignity

Section Two: Philosophical Perspectives of Nature and Human Nature

Outline for Chapter 3: Foundations of Knowing Nature and Human Nature

A. Philosophy of Nature
  1. Seeking a stable source of moral guidance
  2. Other sources of moral guidance
  3. Moving to the knowledge of human nature
B. Forms of Logical Reasoning
  1. Valid logical forms of reasoning
      a. Modus Ponens
      b. Modus Tollens
  2. Invalid logical forms of reasoning
      a. The fallacy of denying the antecedent
      b. The fallacy of affirming the consequent
C. Knowledge of Nature
  1. Nature as the world
  2. Nature as an internal principle
 D. Natural and Artificial
E. Knowledge of Human Nature
  1. An integral union
  2. The dualist perspective
  3. An immaterial source
F. Knowing What Can Be Known in Nature
  1. It is possible to know
      a. invisible capillaries
      b. nature
      c. number

d. statistics
2. Knowing is having universals in the mind
3. Demonstrations on the assumption of the end
G. Stability Within Change
    1. Platonic forms
    2. Aristotelian forms
    3. Living substance is the integral unity of matter energized by form
H. The Known
I. Conclusion
Terminology for Chapter 3
Antecedent
Consequent
Modus Ponens
Modus Tollens
Fallacies
Nature
Artifact
Artificial
Natural
Persistent Vegetative State (PVS)
Substance
Integral union
Matter
Form
Primary matter
Principle of individuation
Principle of stability
Substantial form

Outline for Chapter 4: Humans as Persons in Community

A. Properties of Human Nature
    1.Humans as the knowing subject (knower)
        a. The senses
        b. Human intellectual capacities
        c. The will as appetite
    2. An Excellent Human Life
        a. Respect for others
    3. Characteristic Capacities of Beings
    4. Humans are the Rational Animals
        a. Aquinas on immateriality

Terminology for Chapter 4
Essential
Accidental
Self-transcendence
Outer senses
Inner senses
Cognitive
Estimative
Modally distinct
Intellect
Will
Health
Virtue
Knowing
Percept
Autonomy
Informed consent
Paternalism
Substantiality
Relationality

Section Three: Persons

Outline for Chapter 5: The Practitioner is First a Human Then a Professional

A. Two Ancient Parables
    1.The Ring of Gyges
        a. Justice as a virtue
        b. Pulling this parable forward to our time
        c. Applying lessons from The Ring of Gyges
        d. Virtue of Justice is doing what ought to be done when no one knows it.
    2. The Prodigal Son
        a. Pulling this parable forward to our time
    3. Meaning from the parables
B. Caring for the Self
C. The Healing Act
    1. Culture of integrity
D. The Healing Act as a Moral Act
    1. Sokolowski's Healing Exchange
        a. Expanding Sokolowski's insight of the healing exchange
    2. Informal healer
E. Seedhouse's Exposition of Caring Actions
F. Being Professional
    1. Multifaceted healing practice
    2. The distinction between speculative and practical scientists
G. Conclusion
Terminology for Chapter 5
Integrity
Human act
Moral act
Healing act
Justice
justice
Professional
Caring
Health-care science
Health-care arts

Outline for Chapter 6: The Patient is also a Person

A. The Patient is First a Human Being
B. Vulnerability
    1. Vulnerability follows injury and illness
    2. Vulnerability due to limited freedom
    3. Caregiver vulnerability
    4. Financial and educational vulnerabilities
C. Lessons of Vulnerability
    1. Bonnie and George
    2. Lee Rite
    3. John and Lynne
    4. Defiance makes vulnerable
    5. Laws protect
D. Codes to Protect Human Rights
    1. Human rights are patient rights
E. Laws of Human Nature
F. Being Human as a Foundation for Ethical Standards
    1. Professional codes
    2. Law is an external standard
G. Natural Law Ethics
    1. Eternal law
        a. The expression of eternal law
        b. The expression of eternal law within human life is natural law
    2. Natural Law Ethics Guides Human Life
    3. Human Law
    4. Divine Law
H. Conclusion
Terminology for Chapter 6
Implied consent
Eternal Law
Natural Law
Human Law
Divine Law
Person
Vulnerable
Conscientious objection
Rights and responsibilities

Section Four: Ethical Reasoning and Ethical Theories

Outline for Chapter 7: The Right Action Requires Discernment and Virtue

A. The Need for Virtue
1. The four Cardinal Virtues
2. Six characteristic human responses
3. To see the good and do the good
4. A virtuous action
5. Finding the median
6. A role model
B. Human Excellence
1. The human good
   a. Augustine
   b. Aristotle
C. Ethical Decision Making
1. Reflection grows ethical capacity
2. Practical syllogism
3. Analogical reasoning
4. Ethical analysis
D. Confronting Ethical Dilemmas
1. Listen carefully
   a. Listen to inner self
   b. Listen to situation
   c. Listen to the law, codes, and policies
   d. Listen to the sources of ethical principles
2. Think Clearly
   a. Sorting options as a way of thinking
3. Act with Integrity
E. Sample Case with Ethical Analysis
1. Listen to yourself
2. Listen to the situation
3. Listen to law, codes, and policies
4. Listen to principles
5. Think clearly
6. Check the impact of your actions
7. Apparent options
   a. Covering for J.D. rather than appraising VP of situation
   b. Keeping confidentiality rather than breaking confidentiality
8. Middle ground options

F. Resolving the Ethical Dilemmas
G. Conclusion
Terminology for Chapter 7
Moderation
Wisdom
Courage
Justice
Brute
Vicious
Weak-willed person
Strong-will person
Naturally moral person
Ideal person
Honorable
Beneficial
Legal
Consequentialism
Ethical dilemmas
Analogical reasoning

Outline for Chapter 8: A Short Overview of Philosophical Ethical Perspectives

A. Personal Moral Perspectives
    1. Moral norms are one's personal standards of behavior
    2. Public codes and policies
B. Philosophical Ethical Perspectives
    1. Normative ethics
    2. Universal moral law
    3. Principlism
        a. Nonmaleficence
        b. Beneficence
        c. Autonomy
        d. Justice
    4. Utilitarianism
    5. Ethic of care
C. Conclusion
Terminology for Chapter 8
Morality
Normative
Relativism

Hippocratic tradition
Universal Moral Law
Principlism
Beneficence
Nonmaleficence
Autonomy
Justice
Utilitarianism
Ethic of Care
Hypnotical Imperative
Categorical Imperative

Section Five: Humanity at the Heart of Practice

Outline for Chapter 9: Ethical Issues Related to the Beginning of Life

A. Moral and Legal Accountability
    1. A personal experience
    2. An experience of Socrates
    3. Implied consent
B. Acquiring Protection of Human Rights
    1. When life begins
    2. Defining life
    3. Personhood
    4. Symmetry between the beginning of life and the declaration of death
        a. Cardiac declaration of death
        b. Whole-brain criteria of death
        c. Higher brain death as a criterion
    5. The informed decision
C. Impact of Technology
    1. In-vitro fertilization (IVF)
        a. Moral considerations of IVF include financial and human costs
    2. Cloning
        a. Ethical issues of cloning
    3. Stem Cell Research
D. Conclusion
Terminology for Chapter 9
Self-defense argument
Principle of double effect
Hominization

Individuation
Rationality
Stem cell
Implied consent
Cardiac declaration of death
Whole-brain death
Higher-brain death
Human genome

Outline for Chapter 10: Issues at the End of Life

A. Parameters for Declaring Death
   1. Clinical death
   2. Brain death
   3. A case of brain death following cerebral anoxia
     a. Moral and ethical considerations of this case
     b. Confronting reality
     c. Personal moral decisions
     d. Health-care funding
     e. Practice concerns
   4. Brain death after severe head trauma
   5. When brain death does not occur
   6. The practitioner's role
     a. Judicial intervention
     b. A word of caution
B. Active and Passive Euthanasia
   1. Nutrition and hydration
     a. For organ donors
     b. Neurological deficients
   2. Enhancing life or preventing death
     a. Withholding foods and fluids
     b. Hard Choices for Loving People
     c. Mutual goal setting for supporting families
     d. Comfort care feeding
     e. The last days
   3. Resuscitation
     a. Values and concerns
C. Comfort Care and Letting Die
D. Conclusion

Terminology for Chapter 10
Clinical death
Brain death
Harvard criteria
Persistent or permanent vegetative state (PVS)
Coma
Active euthanasia
Passive euthanasia
Comfort feeding
Decision-making capacity

Outline for Chapter 11: Issues Related to Commitments, Professional Colleagues, Access to Health Care and Institutions

A. The Professionals as Humans
  1. The law
  2. Virtue
  3. As professional
      a. An example from a professional code
      b. Code of Conduct
      c. An example of rules of contact
  4. Integrity in Being and Doing
B. Character and Integrity
  1. Michaud
  2. Virtues which move to action
  3. Integrity
C. Heath Care as a Business
  1. Legal
  2. Beneficial
  3. Honorable
D. Allocation of Scare Resources
  1. Legal
  2. Beneficial
  3. Honorable
  4. Fair distribution requires balance
E. Policies and Gatekeepers
F. Rights and Responsibilities
  1. Natural rights
  2. Civil rights
  3. Rights and responsibilities are reciprocal
G. Conscientious Objections

H. Government Regulations
   1. Health Insurance Portability and Accountability Act of 1196 (HIPAA)
   2. Understanding health information privacy
   3. Equal Employment Opportunity commission (EEOC)
I. Your Rights
   1. Race, color, religion, sex, and national origin
   2. Disability
   3. Age discrimination
   4. Sex discrimination
   5. Sexual harassment
J. Conclusion: Everyday Ethics

Terminology for Chapter 11

Cost/benefit analysis
Equity
Natural rights
Civil rights

APPENDIX C:
TEACHING STRATEGIES

The term "scaffolding" is often used when talking about teaching and learning. First, picture in your mind the scaffolds that are erected outside of a building. The scaffolds hold the workers who are creating or remodeling the structure. With this analogy, the teacher creates and presents learning opportunities that serve as the scaffold, and the students are the builders. The teaching strategies that follow are a few ways in which lessons can be designed to scaffold student learning. These teaching strategies emphasize student-centered learning that encourages the students to be active learners who are building their knowledge. The teacher's role is to be the facilitator of learning, or in other words, the scaffolding.

Think-Pair-Share Discussion Strategy

The teaching strategy known as think-pair-share (TPS) asks students to do each of these three actions within a set time limit. The think aspect often includes the action of reading. You assign a written selection to be read either outside of class or in class. After a short period of time to think about an assigned reading or to read a selected piece, students pair up with a student sitting close to them and discuss what each one thinks about what was read or about the question(s) you have posed.

Pairing encourages conversation. Many times in teacher-led discussions a limited number of students talk. With pairing students for discussions, each person is required to give and receive insights into what is being discussed. This time of sharing with one or two classmates can provide the students clarity and confidence (or thoughtful questions) about what they have read. Students, who may be reluctant to contribute to whole-class discussions, may be more likely to contribute to the later shared discussion after testing their ideas first with a partner. As the facilitator, you will decide the time limit for the pairs' discussions. You will also monitor the paired discussions to extend the time, if discussions are productive, or end the discussions early if students seem to be getting off task.

Finally during the sharing time of TPS, the teacher calls the class together for a review of the paired discussions. The teacher may open the shared discussion by asking, "What are some things that came up in your discussions?" The shared discussion time also gives the teacher an opportunity to clarify any misconceptions, expand the discussion, and/or emphasize key points of the lesson. Again more students may contribute to a shared discussion because they have tried out their ideas first in the paired setting. The goal of TPS is give more students a voice in class discussions.

Teaching an Active Reading Strategy—Read to Share by Color-Coding

Students may say they read an assignment, but they do not remember anything to contribute to class discussions. It may be that these students do not realize that they should read different materials in different ways. If students try to read a textbook as though they were reading a novel for pleasure, they are not reading at the comprehension level needed to succeed in a college course. Students must learn to be active readers, and you can help them by requiring them to color-code a reading assignment.

Color-coding, while reading, slows down students' reading pace and calls for them to make personal connections and classifications while they are reading. For the purpose of this textbook, the following color-coding scheme is suggested:

Yellow Marks thoughts I question or want to discuss
Light green Marks thoughts that impact my life or career
BlueMark thoughts that express my view of the world
EXAMPLE:

An example of a difficult situation was in the news in December 2013 following a California court decision to extend life support for Jahi McMath. The 13 year old girl hemorrhaged after tonsillectomy surgery and went into cardiac arrest. She was resuscitated and put on a ventilator for life support. Three days later she was assessed as brain dead; having no central nervous system function.[1] Thus far, no one has recovered from brain death, so in all fifty states brain dead is dead. The person can be legally taken off of life support and their donated organs transplanted. Jahi's family did not accept this assessment. It is quite natural for her family to think of her as still alive. They could see her chest rise and fall with mechanical ventilation. Cardiac rhythm has been restored so the body has warmth. But, there is no detectable brain activity.

Building Background Knowledge and Front-Loading Vocabulary

Faculty can also support students' reading by building background knowledge and front-loading vocabulary. To do this, teachers give a preview of the important concepts and highlight key vocabulary terms that student will be reading about in the upcoming assignment. This pre-teaching provides a foundation to help students make connections with the new content while they will be reading. Some prior knowledge of key vocabulary makes the reading less of a chore for your students. This is another teaching strategy that encourages students to be active versus passive readers.

Active Learning through Role-play

It is both exciting and rewarding when educators can set the stage and then step back to allow students to take on the task of active learning. Teachers often teach as they were taught, and that may lead to lecture-styled classes. Although the direct teaching style, also known as lecture, can be efficient way to present new information, it may not provide long-lasting content knowledge for students.

Asking student to read scenarios and take on a role can help students become more immersed in classroom discussions. The role-playing can often allow students to shed some inhibitions for speaking out on a topic or to take a side of an argument that the student might not hold himself. The exercises in ethics which follow in Appendix C have been developed and vetted to be used as classroom activities in support of the content form various chapters in the textbook. These activities will support active learning.

APPENDIX D:
CLASSROOM ACTIVITIES LESSON PLANS AND STUDENTS HANDOUTS

The following lesson plans of activities support content from various chapters of this textbook. Student handouts are also included for the activities when necessary. These exercises in ethics include:

1. Values Refugee (for Chapters 1 or 2)
2. The House that Values Built (for Chapters 1 or 2)
3. Reflections on Human Life Activity (for Chapter 3)
4. Take Shelter (Chapters 4 or 8)
5. Ben's Case Study (Chapter 5, 6 or 11)
6. Extension for the Trolley Dilemma (Chapter 8 or as a course review)
7. Generic Cure Hospital (Chapter 11)
8. We Go You Go Bus Company (Chapter 11)

Values Refugee
1. Best used with Chapters 1 or 2
2. Approximate time required for the activity is 30 minutes.
3. Materials list:
   Students need pencil and paper
4. Rationale or statement of purpose for the activity:
   The purpose of this activity is values clarification with particular emphasis on priority setting with the identification of the valuables that can and cannot be compromised. The second half of the activity is concerned with the workplace. It seems that the closer the match between the individual's personal values and the values in the workplace, the greater congruence or comfort the individual will have. With very different values there will be more conflict and tension.
5. Procedures for presenting the activity:
   Tell students the list is for their eyes only. At conclusion, ask students what it was like doing this. Tell them not to talk about

what is on the list, but what was it was like to make the list or how did it felt doing this work.

1. List Valuables
   a. List 13 valuables (values, things, persons—anything that is their valuable). This list is personal and not intended to be shared.
   b. Omit 3, so that 10 remain.
   c. It is hard, but you are a "values refugee" and can only have 5 valuables. Which 5 will you choose for your valuables bag? (This is very difficult for some persons and if they smile or chuckle at the way it is phrased they seem to relax a little, making the selection easier.) They may group valuables, i.e., if they said mother, father, children, they may want to use family.
   d. Rank these 5 valuables from 1-5, 1 being the most important.
   e. Questions
      a. Which of these valuables, if any, would you sacrifice for a good job, actually your dream job?
      b. Which of these valuables, if any, would you sacrifice to save the life of a favorite family member?
      c. Which of these valuables, if any, would you sacrifice to save your own life, in other words, are there some things worth dying for?

B. Workplace
1. Without comment or evaluation, as a group, list on the board valuables in the workplace (business, hospital, information system or organization depending on the focus of the class). This may be 13 or 20 depending on the group.
2. Clump and organize and eliminate until there are only five groupings left. This will usually be something about finances, personnel, quality, reputation, and facilities, (upper management may be included).
3. Ranking these leads to interesting discussion between the relationship between quality service or product and financial stability. I really don't know which is "first." The important thing to me is the way the discussion summarizes much of what they have been learning in business and management courses. And, the way they now see values and a priority of values is a part of the workplace.
6. Wrap-up:
    Ask students to compare the kinds of things on their list and the ones on the board. Ask them to think about a workplace they know. Discuss the need for self-knowledge and congruence between

private and work, or public self.

It is clear that the eliminated valuables are negotiable. They are the grey areas that can be compromised. Some people can compromise all of their inner core valuables and some can compromise none of them. Never judge the students' responses. The purpose is self-awareness. Many times students want to talk about the process and the impact it had on them. It is good to do this.

The House those Values Built

1. Best used with Chapters 1 or 2

It is a follow-up activity to the Values Refugee Activity.

2. Approximate time required for the activity is 20 - 30 minutes.
3. Materials list:

    Student handout (provided at the end of this plan)
4. Rationale or statement of purpose for the activity:

    The purpose of this activity is for students to see that their values determine what principles they see as relevant, and to realize that what they do is a better measure of what they value than what they say. The same holds for all people.

Students may become aware that they have had to sacrifice things they value, like time with their family, to go to school. However, in the end the schooling supports their family and they become role models.

5. Procedures for presenting the activity:
a. Scenario: As a result of your students participation in "The Values Refugee" they have isolated five values. At this time, students will do the activity "The House that Values Built." It is the insight of this activity that values determine principles upon which one will actually act. For example, you may say you value independence, but if you prefer shared assignments you really value interdependence or the anonymity that comes with group work. What one actually does is a better measure of what one values than what a person says.
b. Steps to follow:

    Step 1: Ask the students to list the five values and put them in the basement of a drawing of a house.

    Step2: From each value in the basement, students are asked to create a pillar of principle. For example, if health is a value than the pillar is a healthy life style.

    Step 3: Finally students add an action roof to the drawing. For each principle pillar, the students ask themselves, "What have I done to fulfill this principle?"

Student Handout for The House that Values Built

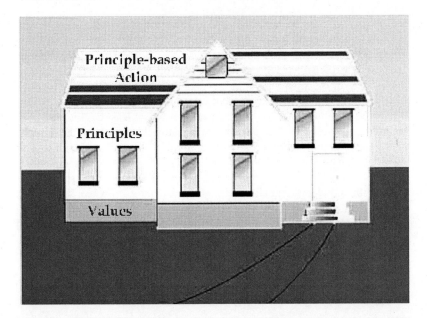

Construct your own house below from the oral directions given to you for this activity.

Self-Reflection Questions for the House that Values Built

Upon completion of your house consider (1) the 'earth' upon which it stands. Of what is it composed? Some have said individuals and society because ethical actions are interpersonal. What do you think? Be fairly specific; don't just repeat individuals and society. Why do you say this?

(2) Take a careful look at the "active roof." To what extent does it actually reflect what you do? Which of these actions have you done today? This week? What are the principles or values behind most of your daily activities?

Your house is a picture of your moral home. Now that you have built your house (your house itself is private) you may want to share with classmates what it was like to do this activity; to identify principles and maybe even having to revise principles to fit what you actually do. What you do reflects the principles you actually accept as important. No one is going to accept that you value playing the piano if you haven't played the piano in a month, unless your arm is in a sling. You value doing your work or caring for family more than piano.

Within this house-building activity and in living decisions, moral actions are principle based actions toward the human good. There are many activities we do every day that we do as living beings that need to sleep, eat, exercise, etc. Moral decisions involve awareness of principles, knowledge of the situation you are facing, and the physical and emotional freedom to make a decision on what would be an excellent human action. There are usually options to be considered, or one at least has the choice of acting or not acting in the situation. A mentally ill person responding to a compulsion is not acting morally or immorally. The designation does not apply. We may note that there is no accountability when the action is not a matter of choice. We are accountable for moral actions because they are done with knowledge and choice.

Reflections on Human Life

1. Best used with Chapter 3.
2. Approximate time required for the activity is 40 - 50 minutes.
3. Materials list:
   Student handout (included at the end of the plan)
4. Rationale or statement of purpose for the activity:
   This activity engages the students in discussion of classic questions in understanding human life. Helping students discover answers is more meaningful than telling them, plus there is not just one answer. The second portion of this exercise develops an awareness of the impact of modern technology on human dignity.
5. Procedures for presenting the activity:
c. Steps to follow:
Divide students into groups of 2 or 3.

First ask student groups to support one of each of the following 3 pairs related to basic questions:

1.1 Human beings are fully explained as biological/social beings subject to evolutionary forces.How do you account for non-material aspects of human life, like two sisters writing e-mail to each other a few minutes apart on the same evening when they haven't written for a few weeks.

OR

1.2 Human beings are not fully explained as biological/social beings subject to evolutionary forces. What evidence do you have that human existence goes beyond the physical and social? What do you consider the other dimension(s)? What supports this answer?

2.1 Dignity accompanies human life (human dignity). It cannot be diminished, taken away or increased in itself.

OR

2.2 Dignity accompanies human life (human dignity), but it can be lost through ones actions and it can be diminished, taken away or increased by the way one is treated.

3.1 Intellectual aspects of human life require an immaterial origin, i.e., from an immaterial being versus parents alone. No one doubts that we come from our parents. Is God required in this generative process?

OR

3.2. An immaterial source is not required in the generation of human life. All humans are biologically generated from their parents

Then ask student to mark these listed technologies by the following criteria: The goal is to make clear which of the following makes richer the way that we perceive and value fellow humans? Use a CHECK behind those that increase the perceived value of a human life. Use an "X" behind those that decrease the perceived value of a human life. Provide a short explanation of each answer.

Television, cable and streaming video
Telephone
Cell phone and Skype
Internet
Sexually explicit tapes and videos
Diagnostic sonograms
Sonograms of embryos
Universal Declaration of Human Rights
Helsinki accords
Chemical Contraception
Barrier contraception for preventing STD and HIV transmission
Abortion
Cloning
Genome editing for disease prevention
Genome editing for attribute selection
Embryonic Stem Cell Research
IVF for infertile couples
IVF with sperm donor for single women
Adoption of a child
Death penalty
Military action to restore peace

Put C in front of each of the above that make human life a commodity, places a monetary value?

Remember to provide a short explanation of each answer and defend whether this has a positive or negative impact on our perception of human dignity, and why?

    d. Expectations from participants or groups of participants. This
       activity could provide a submission for grading based on
       thoughtfulness.
6. Wrap-up or "take-away" from the activity:
Increased awareness of the uniqueness of human life and how
actual value and perception is changed by modern technology.

See the next page for the student handout.

Student Handout for Reflection on Human Life

A. Support one of each of the following 3 pairs:
1.1 Human beings are fully explained as biological/social beings subject to evolutionary forces.How do you account for non-material aspects of human life, like two sisters writing e-mail to each other a few minutes apart on the same evening when they haven't written for a few weeks.
   OR
1.2 Human beings are not fully explained as biological/social beings subject to evolutionary forces. What evidence do you have that human existence goes beyond the physical and social? What do you consider the other dimension(s)? What supports this answer?

2.1 Dignity accompanies human life (human dignity). It cannot be diminished, taken away or increased in itself.
   OR
2.2 Dignity accompanies human life (human dignity), but it can be lost through ones actions and it can be diminished, taken away or increased by the way one is treated.

3.1 Intellectual aspects of human life require an immaterial origin, i.e., from an immaterial being versus parents alone. No one doubts that we come from our parents. Is God required in this generative process?
   OR
3.2. An immaterial source is not required in the generation of human life. All humans are biologically generated from their parents

B. Which of the following increase the way that we perceive and value fellow humans? Use a CHECK behind those that increase the perceived value of a human life. Use an "X" behind those that decrease the perceived value of a human life. Provide a short explanation of each answer.

   Television
   Telephone
   Cell phone and Skype
   Internet
   Pornography
   Sonograms
   Universal Declaration of Human Rights
   Helsinki accords

Contraception
Barrier contraception for STD illness of a partner
Abortion
Embryonic Stem Cell Research
IVF for infertile couples
IVF with Sperm donor for single women
Adoption of a child
Death penalty
Military action to restore peace

Put C in front of each of the above that make human life a commodity, places a monetary value? Provide a short explanation of each answer and defend whether this is positive or negative and why?

If you hold human dignity can be altered, explain the impact of each of the above on human dignity?

Take Shelter
1. Best used with Chapter 4 or 8.
2. Approximate time required for the activity is 50 minutes.
3. Materials list:
   Student handout (provided at the end of this plan)
   White board in classroom or poster paper
4. Statement of purpose for the activity:
   This activity enables students to see there are many preferences that become prejudices when they are the basis for decision-making. It also has students experience group decision-making under pressure.
5. Procedures for presenting the activity:

Scenario: Your group is called Command Central, and it is a division of the United Nations Research Center on Communal Living. There are 12 research centers around the world. Members of the communes agree that Command Central will decide who enters an emergency shelter if there is not room for everyone. This is to avoid possible conflict among commune members.

Word has been received that a commune in the Aleutian Islands off the coast of Alaska, USA, is endangered by lava flow. The island compound will be completely submerged in lava. No one thought this would ever happen as the volcano has been silent for over a century, but there was a massive northeast earthquake this morning. Unfortunately, the commune has grown to 10 persons while there are only sufficient supplies (food, water, and adequate fresh air flow) in the emergency shelter for 6 persons for 3 months. The shelter is not expected to be accessed for 3 months while the lava cools and the entrance is discovered.

In 25 minutes, your Command Central group must provide **a unanimous decision** of who will and will not enter the shelter, along with reasons for these decisions. Reasons are required for the report which will be filed. If 6 persons are not chosen to go into the shelter within 25 minutes, all persons will be lost in the flood of red hot lava.

    a. Divide the class into groups of 4 or 5 students.
    b. Give students the handouts. Make sure students know they have a 25-minute time limit. However if all groups decide sooner, feel free to move onto the reporting phase of the activity.

c. While student groups are working, construct a recording grid on a white board or poster paper that has 10 columns and rows that equal the number of groups.

	scientist	wife	TV host	medical student	acct.	priest	football handyman	robot	majorette	lawyer
Group1										
Group2										

At the end of the time limit, have each recorder put an "X" in the column of the members **who will not** be going into the shelter as determined by their group. Hold off discussing reasons for the groups' decisions until the grid is completed with each group's report.

Once all persons are recorded make a short note by each person that captures why that person was selected to enter the shelter or not.

d. Begin the discussion of reasons. Note the negative biases of age, alcoholism, and lack of utility and the positive biases of education, age, and utility that may surface from the reasons given for a person being excluded or included into the shelter. Draw attention to the idea that personal biases when used for decision making are also known as prejudices.

6. Wrap-up:

At the conclusion of the discussion, explore a more ethical way of deciding who will enter the shelter by drawing straws rather than deciding on stereotypes. Select ten students to represent the members of the Aleutian commune and have them draw straws. Discuss the experience of being included or excluded.

See the next page for the student handout.

Student Handout for Take Shelter

Your group is called Command Central, and it is a division of the United Nations Research Center on Communal Living. There are 12 research centers around the world. Members of the communes agree that Command Central will decide who enters an emergency shelter if there is not room for everyone. This is to avoid possible conflict among commune members.

Word has been received that a commune in the Aleutian Islands off the coast of Alaska, USA, is endangered by lava flow. Within half an hour, the island compound will be completely submerged in lava. No one thought this would ever happen as the volcano has been silent for over a century, but there was a massive northeast earthquake this morning. Unfortunately, the commune has grown to 10 persons while there are only sufficient supplies (food, water, and adequate fresh air flow) in the emergency shelter for 6 persons for 3 months. The shelter is not expected to be accessed for 3 months while the lava cools and the entrance is discovered.

In 25 minutes, your Command Central group must provide **a unanimous decision** of who will and will not enter the shelter, along with reasons for these decisions. Reasons are required for the report which will be filed. If 6 persons are not chosen to go into the shelter within a half hour, all persons will be lost in the flood of red hot lava.

You have been given the Aleutian file with the following brief descriptions. The decision must be unanimous and will be permanent once reported. Your group needs to determine a recorder and reporter. These two positions may be held by the same person, but separate persons are preferable.

Current residents of the Aleutian Island Commune include:

1. Scientist who is conducting adaptation experiments in the Aleutian biosphere.
2. The scientist's wife who is three months pregnant.
3. TV celebrity taping a show on-site for the week.
4. Third-year medical student on a public health visit.
5. Accountant who just finished college and recently joined the commune.
6. An alcoholic Anglican priest.
7. A former professional football player who serves the commune as handyman for repairs.
8. Robot for domestic duties.
9. A high school majorette visiting for the semester.

10. A Washington DC lawyer studying liability issues.

Decide individually which persons you want to recommend go in the lava shelter. Then share your individual decisions as a way to start to determine who will enter the shelter and why. Remember, this must be a unanimous decision. Be sure to record your answers of whom and why each person is selected to enter the shelter. A full report will be expected at the end of the 25 minutes.

Ben's Case Study

1. Best used with Chapter 6 or 11
2. Approximate time required for the activity is 40 -50 minutes.
3. Materials list:
   Student handout (provided at the end of this plan. See it for detailed questions sets.)
4. Rationale or statement of purpose for the activity:
   This activity provides the opportunity for the student to consider the impact of acting on their own values without notifying a supervisor of a problem. And for the student to realize the importance of working with administration to make changes that benefit all patients.
5. Procedures for presenting the activity:
   Scenario: Ben works as a technologist in x-ray special exams for a large inner city hospital. The hospital is in financial difficulty, so administration decided to use less expensive kidney dye on the uninsured patients, most of whom are homeless street persons. These patients represent 30 – 40 % of the hospital's clientele. Ben observed that patients had more frequent and more severe adverse reactions from the cheaper dye. Feeling that all patients deserve quality care, he decided to not follow the administrative order and used the best dye on everyone. He did not tell anyone what he was doing. He was able to go into the supply room and take the dye he needed without detection. He put the required solution on the patient's record but used the better product. Ben felt justified in what he was doing. He reasoned, the hospital was using an unfair practice. Additionally, it was just money for the hospital. For these poor patients it meant a difference in suffering and possibly even death.
   Steps to follow:
   Have students respond **to ONE (1)** of the **question sets in the student handout** and have students presume one of the roles. There is wide latitude for students to frame the ethical questions from a position in the scenario. Remind students to be creative in adding details to the scenario as needed.
6. Expectations from participants or groups of participants:
   Require students to identify a personal moral statement and to apply course content throughout their work.

Student Handout for Ben's Case Study

Scenario: Ben works as a technologist in x-ray special exams for a large inner city hospital. The hospital is in financial difficulty, so administration decided to use less expensive kidney dye on the uninsured patients, most of whom are homeless street persons. These patients represent 30 – 40 % of the hospital's clientele. Ben observed that patients had more frequent and more severe adverse reactions from the cheaper dye. Feeling that all patients deserve quality care, he decided to not follow the administrative order and used the best dye on everyone. He did not tell anyone what he was doing. He was able to go into the supply room and take the dye he needed without detection. He put the required solution on the patient's record but used the better product. Ben felt justified in what he was doing. He reasoned, the hospital was using an unfair practice. Additionally, it was just money for the hospital. For these poor patients it meant a difference in suffering and possibly even death.

Please respond **to ONE (1)** of the following question sets. Presume the role you want to take. There is wide latitude for you to frame the ethical questions from your position in the scenario. Do not be afraid to be creative in adding to your scenario the detail you need. Be sure I can identify your personal moral statement. **Apply course content throughout your work.**

1. Evaluate the ruling made by hospital administration in terms of policy development, financial management and in terms of virtue and respect for persons. Support your discussion and provide an alternative solution from your **personal** and **professional** ethical content. *You are Ben's supervisor.*

2. Evaluate patient responsibility, without insurance on what basis are patients entitled to care? Answer for both A. the employed underinsured; and, B. the indigent poor who will never pay. Within this last group are the patients Ben is concerned about. Support your discussion from your **personal** and **professional** ethical content. *You are a patient advocate.*

3. Evaluate Ben's reasoning and actions. If you agree with his decision and actions support your position from your **personal** and **professional** ethical content. If you disagree with his decision and actions explain this and offer an alternative. Support your answers from your **personal** and **professional** ethical content. *You are a clinician caring for the same patients as Ben.*

4. As a teacher of ethics confronted with a student revealing this

situation on a student report, decide what needs to be done based on a careful analysis of the situation and your role as a teacher? Support your discussion from your **personal** and **professional** ethical content. *You are Ben's Business Ethic's teacher.*

5. *From the perspective of hospital security,* address the hospital's responsibility to provide a secure environment. There is currently an open policy with supplies that trusts clinical employees to only take what they need. They are expected to sign for supplies used. Support your discussion from your **personal** and **professional** ethical content.

You are an officer at the hospital. Ought there to be a report to metropolitan police? How would that impact the hospital?

Extension Activity for the Trolley Dilemma
1. Best used with Chapter 8 or as a course review.
2. Approximate time required for the activity is 50 minutes.
3. Materials list:
   Student handout (included at the end of this plan)
4. Rationale or statement of purpose for the activity:
   The trolley dilemma is a well-known thought problem developed by British philosopher Philippa Foot in 1967.
5. Procedures for presenting the activity (See student handout for full details):
   Present the trolley dilemma first and by itself. After discussion of the trolley scenario, move to the transplant scenario with the surgeon's decision.

Scenario Part 1:
Suppose you are the driver of a trolley whose brakes have just failed. On the track ahead of you are five people; the banks are so steep that they will not be able to get off the track in time. The track has a spur leading off to the right, and you can turn the trolley onto it. Unfortunately there is a trolley engineer doing an inspection on the right-hand track. You can turn the trolley, killing the engineer; or you can refrain from turning the trolley, and the five will die.

Step 1—Ask students to discuss the scenario with other classmates. Let everyone share their ideas and prepare a report for the class that may be submitted for graded class credit. Thoughtfully consider the following situation. Provide your own ideas and a thoughtful consideration of Natural Law and Virtue Ethics (be sure to include descriptions of the ethical perspectives).

As the instructor, you may prefer to focus on selected frameworks you wish the students to consider.

Scenario Part 2:
You are a great transplant surgeon. Five of your patients need new organs - one needs a new heart, the others need, respectively, liver, stomach, spleen, and spinal cord. All of these patients are of the same, relatively rare, blood-type. By chance, you learn of a healthy specimen with that very blood-type. You can take the healthy specimen's parts, killing him, and install them in your patients, potentially saving them. Or, you can refrain from taking the healthy specimen's parts, potentially letting your patient's die.

Step 2—Again ask students to discuss the scenario with other classmates. Let everyone share their ideas and prepare a report for the class that may be submitted for graded class credit. Thoughtfully consider the following situation. Provide your own ideas and a thoughtful consideration of Natural Law and Virtue Ethics (be sure to include descriptions of the ethical perspectives).

6. Expectations from participants or groups of participants:
   The goal of the written reports is to provide more awareness of the ethical frameworks.

Student Handout for Trolley Dilemma Extended

Please discuss the following scenario with classmates. Let everyone share their ideas and prepare a report for the class that can be submitted for **graded class credit.** Thoughtfully consider the following situation. Provide your own ideas and a thoughtful consideration of Natural Law and Virtue Ethics (be sure to include descriptions of the ethical perspectives). **The goal of this paper is to provide more awareness of the ethical frameworks.**

A. Suppose you are the driver of a trolley whose brakes have just failed. On the track ahead of you are five people; the banks are so steep that they will not be able to get off the track in time. The track has a spur leading off to the right, and you can turn the trolley onto it. Unfortunately there is a trolley engineer doing an inspection on the right-hand track. You can turn the trolley, killing the engineer; or you can refrain from turning the trolley, and the five will die.

Questions:
1. Is it morally permissible for you to turn the trolley? Why or why not?
2. Consider the distinction between letting die and killing.
3. Consider accountability and responsibility of each person involved.
4. After providing a solution as discussed by your group, use natural law and virtue ethics to provide philosophically considered positions.
5. Would it make a difference in how you present your position if the person on the single track was (a) your best friend or (b) your child? (c) yourself?

Now consider a second scenario.

Again discuss the scenario with classmates. Let everyone share their ideas and prepare a report for the class that can be submitted for **graded class credit**. Thoughtfully consider the following situation. Provide your own ideas and a thoughtful consideration of Natural Law and Virtue Ethics (be sure to include descriptions of the ethical perspectives). **The goal of this paper is to provide more awareness of the ethical frameworks.**

B. You are a great transplant surgeon. Five of your patients need new organs - one needs a new heart, the others need, respectively, liver, stomach, spleen, and spinal cord. All of these patients are of the same, relatively rare, blood-type. By chance, you learn of a healthy specimen with that very blood-type. You can take the healthy specimen's parts, killing him, and install them in your patients, potentially saving them. Or, you can refrain from taking the healthy specimen's parts, potentially letting your patient's die.

Similar Questions:
1. Is it morally permissible for you to take the healthy person's organs? Why or Why not?
2. Consider the distinction between letting die and killing
3. Consider accountability and responsibility of each person involved.
4. After providing a solution as discussed by your group, use natural law and virtue ethics to provide philosophically considered positions. (3 positions required)
5. Would it make a difference in how you present your position if the healthy person was (a) your best friend or (b) your child? (c) yourself?

Additional Question: What are the moral differences between these two cases? Explain using **theoretical** and personal content.

Generic Cure Hospital

1. Best used with Chapter 11.

   It is also possible to use this activity as a review of ethics. The scenario presents the seven most common ethical perspectives through the roles of the committee members. This activity is usually used on or just before the last class so students have familiarity with ethical content.

2. Approximate time required for the activity is 50 minutes.

   Assigning the students to read the hand-out materials ahead of the activity encourages thoughtfulness and independent decision making. However, this activity has been successful with students reading it for the first time at the time of the activity.

3. Materials list:

   Student hand-out (provided at the end of this plan)

4. Statement of purpose for the activity:

   This activity gives students the opportunity to become aware of a diversity views. Students may solve the situation quite simply with cultural and family values, but professional clinicians need to utilize philosophical principles. This activity also allows students to practice respecting views different from their own. While it was written for participants of health-care management curricula, reflective learning has resulted for a wide variety of persons in the inter-disciplinary, undergraduate classroom.

5. Procedures for presenting the activity:

   Scenario: The scenario is set at a fictitious, local not-for-profit hospital. There is limited information given about the hospital so that students have maximum opportunity to identify with it and to prevent the assumption that they know the location. Students will each assume a role as one member of the hospital's ethics committee.

   Cases: There are five brief cases on the student hand-out. The brevity is purposeful as it allows students to identify with similar cases in their own experiences. An abbreviated version of the cases, each with a short rationale given in bold text, follows:

   1. A free-standing fertility organization wishes to use the hospital's outpatient facilities. **The desired focus of discussion in this situation is an institution's rights and responsibilities when entering a contract. It is also a less threatening way of addressing the value of human life at its beginning rather**

than the abortion issue. It is suggested to shy away from this polarizing question.

2. A physician admits a patient for radiation therapy, but the patient is also on a non-FDA approved therapy. **This case brings up patient and caregiver rights and responsibilities and the autonomy of both persons. It also allows a look at standard and alternative therapies and the legal criterion of "usual and customary interventions."**

3. From circumstances, it appears that a nurse is practicing euthanasia. **This case points to the need for further assessment and management's responsibility to protect patients, staff, and the hospital itself. It may also lead to discussions on euthanasia, although that is not the focus topic here.**

4. A near-by community hospital is closing. Generic Cure has been asked to markedly increase its charity services. **This item looks at the clash between altruism and fiscal responsibilities. It also addresses the question of who receives care; is the right to care derived from being a human being or from being a member of society**

   e. Students will be put into randomized groups of 4 to 7 depending on class size.

   f. Students will establish committee membership; designate a chairperson (usually administration or physician), a recording secretary, and an agenda.

   g. Background information for each case:

1. The ethics committee decided to ask the fertility organization to propose a contract. One of the items desired was that mothers were expected to deliver at the hospital. The concerns of the religious member were ignored and the member was viewed as someone pushing religion. The politically powerful members felt that requesting the contract would probably squelch the issue.

2. A potential solution from the committee included having the doctor give the injections. However, since the drug was not approved, this was still problematic. All agreed that the nurses could not give the injections and put their licenses at risk. Shockingly, since the committee did not want to loose favor with Dr. Q., they recommended he loose privileges until he brought his records up to date. He was in violation of hospital policy with his charting being 6 months behind. The committee gave him no answer on the Laetrile.

3. Case 3 is adapted from a widely known case of a nurse believed to be injecting potassium chloride into terminally ill patients. She was never convicted, and was last known to be doing wellness physicals for an insurance company.

An important aspect of case 3 is that the nurse cannot be placed on administrative leave if the hospital wants to uncover what is happening. Additionally, to place her on leave is to open the potential of a law suit. The case makes the husband the coroner as a way to close the simple solution of autopsies, which would not tell who the responsible party was. Lastly, it is interesting to note that patients often die on the night shift when metabolism drops. It can also happen if the evening nurse did not give adequate pain coverage so when the night staff came on, they had to medicate everyone. If one waits a long time for medication, it takes more medication to bring pain relief. This makes it look like the night nurse has a problem when actually the evening nurse, being afraid to medicate, is the problem.

4. The overall point of case 4 is that even if a hospital facility is philanthropic, it must maintain solvency. This case also brings up the reciprocal nature of rights and responsibilities. Students often suggest fundraising to establish a fund for indigent care or asking more hospitals to assist with such care

6. Wrap-up:

To facilitate a whole-class discussion, have the recording secretary for each group read the statement of suggestions and the rationale for a case. The discussion of all four cases may run longer than one class period, so it is suggested to take one case at a time to allow for carry over to another day.

See the next page for the student handout.

Student Hand-out for the Generic Cure Hospital

The Generic Cure Hospital
Management Ethics Committee Meeting

Generic Cure hospital is a not-for-profit hospital which reinvests its earnings into equipment, patient services, and assisting other not-for-profit organizations. The physician founder-directors are on salary. The hospital was opened twelve years ago to meet the need for these university-based physicians to have a place for private practice.

You are one member of the hospital's ethics committee. The committee is to provide guidance to hospital professionals who must make difficult decisions.

In order to have a quorum, at least four of the following members need to be present. You will role-play as one of the following committee members. In parenthesis you will find the point of view you will portray for the committee member. Select from the following:

1. **Community member**—on the Board of Trustees of a local bank (wants to ensure that actual benefits to the community outweigh the social costs –internal and external costs of an action)
2. **Religious member**—not associated with the hospital (concerned with the will of God)
3. **Physician on staff**—paid hospital employee (concerned with professional standards and behaviors required by the professional doctor-patient relationship)
4. **Member of administration**—paid hospital employee (concerned with policy and contract rights and duties)
5. **Social worker**—(concerned that autonomy and individual values are given priority)
6. **Nurse**—paid hospital employee (concerned with healing, health promotion, and treating persons with respect)
7. **Medical records librarian**—paid hospital employee (concerned with policy requirements and privacy issues)

Expected Outcomes
1. As a committee you will meet to first establish (1) committee membership, (2) a chairperson—usually administration or physician, (3)a recording secretary, and (4) an agenda.

2. Discuss the cases and make suggestions, from your role on the committee, to assist those responsible for making the decisions in each case.
3. The recording secretary will prepare a statement of suggestions and rationale that will be reported to the larger group during class discussions.
4. The following questions may assist your committee's work:
a. What are the ethical issues versus financial, managerial, and/or communication issues involved in the case?
b. What are the values or principles in conflict, if any?
c. What additional information or clarifications are needed?
d. Whose rights and responsibilities are involved?
e. Who is entitled to make the decision?
f. Is there legal guidance?
g. What is the honorable solution?
h. What action(s) would be beneficial?
i. What guidance can be offered by the committee?

There are five brief cases. The brevity is purposeful as it allows you to identify with similar cases in from your own experiences. The case topics are as follows:

1. A free-standing fertility organization wishes to use the hospital's outpatient facilities.
2. A physician admits a patient for radiation therapy, but the patient is also on a non-FDA approved therapy.
3. From circumstances, it appears that a nurse is practicing euthanasia.
4. A dependable, long-term employee in a critical hospital position blames his recent payroll errors on his illness (AIDS).
5. A near-by community hospital is closing. Generic Cure has been asked to markedly increase its charity services.

You-Go-We-Go Bus Company

1. Best used with Chapter 11.
2. Approximate time required for the activity is 90 minutes. This full activity takes about 1 ½ hours. To use less time omit step two and say the meeting will be in 35 minutes.
3. Materials list:
   Student handout (provided at the end of this plan)
4. Rationale for the activity:
   Consideration of options for setting priorities. Use of EEOC and non-discrimination.
5. Procedures for presenting the activity:
   Scenario: Six months ago your franchise purchased this newly developed suburban mass transit company from its original owner and developer. You run this division of 50 buses and approximately 39 full and part-time personnel (drivers are part-time split shift workers). There is a very tight budget.

Steps to follow:

Step 1: You now need to determine which the essential positions are and who will fill them. You may combine positions: (1) general and financial manager of the franchise, (2) personnel manager, (3) accountant/payroll manager,(4) office and parts department manager, (5) service manager for those who takes care of the buses mechanically and electronically, (6) scheduler for drivers and custodial personnel, (7) driver and union representative.

Step 2: The mother company prefers a participative management style within its franchises. Write down who is filling which positions and develop a chart showing the lines of authority (a flow chart) reflecting the We-Go-You-Go Bus Company's management.

The mission of the company is to provide customer oriented, safe, convenient, and affordable bus service that will supplement and connect with the municipal bus services.

Prepare a logo reflecting your management team and mission.

These first steps are designed to help participants identify with their franchise and their place within the business community.

Step 3: Although you bought the franchise six months ago, the company has been operating successfully for 2 years and enjoys a good reputation. Very shortly you are having a general management meeting (with employee and union representation) to resolve some problems. Read over the following items to be discussed and establish an agenda based on priority. **Support your choices for the agenda and solutions from ethical as well as business principles.**

There are two rather natural priorities, safety-picking up on the mission, and financial, potential cost to the company. Some groups have prioritized based on projected time required to resolve the item during the meeting. All are reasonable, although I think a case can be made for safety. My goal was for students to grapple with "how to decide."

Step 4: Meeting: Each person participates in each case from the business position they fulfill, if information is needed but not on this page, you may ask or develop it. **Prepare solutions and reasons for the solutions selected by your company from ethical and business principles.**

It is expected that business students will look to virtue and the business model of the text, legal, honorable, and beneficial.

Step 5: In about 35 to 60 minutes, a member of the mother company will be here to receive and discuss your report, including logo, lines of authority, agenda rationale and ethical responses to the following situations that have surfaced in the last 6 months. These actually occurred at a real bus company at a major US city within a 6 month period. If working with a 50 minute class, assign the reading and company development in the preceding class or between classes as homework.

The solutions of the actual company are included in these bold italics written after the agenda items. A few years ago the company was thriving.

Agenda items:
1. Mr. David Jones, assistant to the payroll manager since the company was founded submitted a letter of resignation three weeks ago with termination due this week. He has been a stable and dependable employee. His work record was good until recently. In the last three to four weeks he has been sullen and had 4 personal leave days. When he submitted his letter he said he had left his wife and wanted to move to another town. He values his work and doesn't want to leave abruptly but he feels he must leave because during one of their arguments he hit his wife and she is pressing charges.

Mr. Jones came to the personnel office earlier this week and requested to withdraw his letter of resignation. His wife dropped charges and he has decided not to move. Someone has been hired to fill his position. They have not yet been trained for the position. Should the company honor his request or ask that he resign as originally intended considering that he is still going to be involved in a potentially draining divorce proceeding? The company cannot afford payroll errors. What should be done, how can this be resolved?

The company felt they had to honor the contract to hire the new person as legally binding and invited the gentleman we are calling Mr. Jones to apply for the next available opening. They would rehire him and would not be prejudiced by his personal life. It is necessary to stay with employment behaviors. I have many women who would not let him back into the company and some men: an interesting point of discussion.

2. Mike has been doing repairs on buses for 15 years and has been affiliated with the current *service manager* in different shops for 10 years. He is an excellent mechanic and has kept buses on the road by improvising when the company had no money to buy needed new equipment. Nevertheless, the new equipment which has been purchased in the last year has electronic parts and Mike has made several installation mistakes. He has never read the manuals that came with the new electronic equipment and he just doesn't seem to have grasped how they work. He gets defensive when asked about the new technology by the *service manager* he has known for 10 years. It is suspected that he cannot read but, with strong expressions, he claims that he can and that the *service manager* is prejudiced. The service manager is requesting recommendations. He is concerned for public safety and he wants to protect Mike from making an error that would endanger the riders as this would result in an automatic dismissal according to company policies. Manufacturers no longer contribute engines and parts to training schools and with the new electronics many schools have closed. There is no employee assistance program. It may be necessary to ask him to leave but, if so, you must be able to answer to the union.

Important points are that one cannot discriminate against Mike for a learning disability. My impression is that he cannot be the only employee tested. Some students suggest dividing up mechanical duties between those jobs requiring computer ability and those who do not. The parts manager could order for those doing mechanical duties. After what is usually a lively discussion, I share that one morning a driver ran a bus into the building at slow speed; Mike had put the brakes on backwards. Mike has done brakes for 15 years. One can only think he was under excessive stress. I call this a management failure.

3. Last week the company was cited by the EPA for contaminating the environment with oil. There is a small ditch on the down side of the

bus lot. There is a 15 degree slope toward the ditch. This is just enough so that oil drains into the ditch from the parked buses. It is normal and unavoidable that buses leak slightly. It had never occurred to administration that this little ditch fed into a bigger one and on into the river. The city provided this land. The 50 buses barely fit on the lot.

The citation was a warning. However if the situation is not corrected, the fine is $1,000,000 or more. The ideal solution is to build a reservoir and process the water so there is no oil in it. This would cost nearly $1,200,000.

The office and parts manager suggested removable pans that could be drained into a recycle bin, but the service manager is concerned drivers would just run over them spilling accumulated oil and making the drivers responsible for the company problems. Since last week one of the cleaning people has been working full time to put down absorbent and clean up the oil every day before the rain can wash it into the ditch. **A long term solution is needed.**

Since the city gave the land, it is interesting to speculate if the city carries any responsibility. The company decided they did and requested the city provide a more appropriate site. After about a year they did so. Until a new site was provided, the company continued the short term solution.

The company opted to continue the short term solution before knowing they would receive land. From students in military, I understand the Air Force controls the inevitable oil leak through a drip pan placed on landing and removed for flight.

4. Last month materials came from OSHA about the new law for infectious disease control that goes into effect the first of the year. Hepatitis non-A non-B is a special strain of virus that often results in death. It is acquired through contact with contaminated body fluids, like blood and vomit. If the company fully complies with the law and trains all personnel there will be a tremendous outlay of money. Each set of Hepatitis non-A non-B injections costs $150. The film costs $500. In addition there is money spent on salaries and extra coverage during training sessions which could also mean overtime pay.

You need to decide who needs training and how to manage the cost-benefit ratio, i.e. should you buy the film or share it with other companies in the area? Should you ignore the requirement and hope to not get investigated? How can you decide and what should be done? OSHA believes transit personnel are at risk even though your drivers report an incidence of vomiting or injury about once every six months.

The company opted to begin inoculations with the drivers because they are most likely to be exposed. In a surprising disclosure it was learned the drivers clean the buses. Since they are short on funds, they do not have cleaning people. The company decided to buy the film so it will be available whenever they can organize some staff to view it. What OSHA requires is a plan, not a completed project, so as long as the company is in process of fulfilling requirements they are okay.

5. At a recent workshop for the mass transit industry, workman's compensation cases were discussed. Lately 3 persons filed and won compensation for heart attacks on the basis of their having a high stress job. This was in spite of the fact that they participated in high risk behaviors like smoking and drinking a lot of coffee. These were all top level managers and were very productive and creative people.

The parent company is concerned because of the steep rise in workman's compensation insurance and because the public relations manager of the parent company had a heart attack last year. For a while there was reportedly careful diet compliance and no smoking but recently these behaviors have returned. The top administrators of the parent company are considering finding a way to force resignation of this public relations manager. Your division has been asked to file a confidential report of agreement or non-agreement to the forced retirement and why you hold that position.

This provides an opportunity to realize that nothing stays confidential. The persons involved decided not to respond at all, hoping higher management would calm down and the request would "blow over," which it did. We also talk about what to do with a politically "outrageous" request that carries risk to the franchised company no matter what you respond.

Student Handout for We-Go-You-Go Bus Company

Step one. Six months ago your franchise purchased this newly developed suburban mass transit company from its original owner and developer. You run this division of 50 buses and approximately 39 full and part-time personnel (drivers are part-time split shift workers). There is a very tight budget. **You now need to determine which the essential positions are and who will fill them.** You may combine positions: 1. general and financial manager of the franchise, 2. personnel manager, 3. accountant/payroll manager, 4. office and parts department manager, 5. service manager for those who takes care of the buses mechanically and electronically, 6. scheduler for drivers and custodial personnel, 7. driver and union representative.

Step two. The mother company prefers a participative management style within its franchises. Write down who is filling which positions and develop a chart showing the lines of authority (a flow chart) reflecting the We Go You Go Bus Company's management.

The mission of the company is to provide customer oriented, safe, convenient, and affordable bus service that will supplement and connect with the municipal bus services.

Prepare a logo reflecting your management team and mission.

Step three. Although you bought the franchise six months ago, the company has been operating successfully for 2 years and enjoys a good reputation. Very shortly you are having a general management meeting (with employee and union representation) to resolve some problems. Read over the following items to be discussed and establish an agenda based on priority. **Support your choices for the agenda and solutions from ethical as well as business principles.**

Step four. Meeting: Each person participates in each case from the business position they fulfill, if information is needed but not on this page, you may ask or develop it. **Prepare solutions and reasons for the solutions selected by your company from ethical and business principles.**

Step five.
In about 45 to 60 minutes, a member of the mother company will be here to receive and discuss your report, including logo, lines of authority, and agenda rationale and ethical responses to the following situations that

have surfaced in the last 6 months. These actually occurred at a real bus company at a major US city within a 6 month period.

Agenda items:

1. Mr. David Jones, assistant to the payroll manager since the company was founded submitted a letter of resignation three weeks ago with termination due this week. He has been a stable and dependable employee. His work record was good until recently. In the last three to four weeks he has been sullen and had 4 personal leave days. When he submitted his letter he said he had left his wife and wanted to move to another town. He values his work and doesn't want to leave abruptly but he feels he must leave because during one of their arguments he hit his wife and she is pressing charges.

Mr. Jones came to the personnel office earlier this week and requested to withdraw his letter of resignation. His wife dropped charges and he has decided not to move. Someone has been hired to fill his position. They have not yet been trained for the position. Should the company honor his request or ask that he resign as originally intended considering that he is still going to be involved in a potentially draining divorce proceeding? The company cannot afford payroll errors. What should be done, how can this be resolved?

2. Mike has been doing repairs on buses for 15 years and has been affiliated with the current service manager in different shops for 10 years. He is an excellent mechanic and has kept buses on the road by improvising when the company had no money to buy needed new equipment. Nevertheless, the new equipment which has been purchased in the last year has electronic parts and Mike has made several installation mistakes. He has never read the manuals that came with the new electronic equipment and he just doesn't seem to have grasped how they work. He gets defensive when asked about the new technology by the service manager he has known for 10 years. It is suspected that he cannot read but, with strong expressions, he claims that he can and that the service manager is prejudiced. The service manager is requesting recommendations. He is concerned for public safety and he wants to protect Mike from making an error that would endanger the riders as this would result in an automatic dismissal according to company policies. Manufacturers no longer contribute engines and parts to training schools and with the new electronics many schools have closed. There is no employee assistance program. It may be necessary to ask him to leave but, if so, you must be able to answer to the union.

3. Last week the company was cited by the EPA for contaminating the environment with oil. There is a small ditch on the down side of the bus lot. There is a 15 degree slope toward the ditch. This is just enough so that oil drains into the ditch from the parked buses. It is normal and unavoidable that buses leak slightly. It had never occurred to administration that this little ditch fed into a bigger one and on into the river. The city provided this land. The 50 buses barely fit on the lot.

The citation was a warning, but if the situation is not corrected the fine is $1,000,000 or more. The ideal solution is to build a reservoir and process the water so there is no oil in it. This would cost nearly $1,200,000.

The office and parts manager suggested removable pans that could be drained into a recycle bin, but the service manager is concerned drivers would just run over them spilling accumulated oil and making the drivers responsible for the company problems. Since last week one of the cleaning people has been working full time to put down absorbent and clean up the oil every day before the rain can wash it into the ditch. **A long term solution is needed.**

4. Last month materials came from OSHA about the new law for infectious disease control that goes into effect the first of the year. Hepatitis non-A non-B is a special strain of virus that often results in death. It is acquired through contact with contaminated body fluids, like blood and vomit. If the company fully complies with the law and trains all personnel there will be a tremendous outlay of money. Each set of Hepatitis non-A non-B injections costs $150. The film costs $500. In addition there is money spent on salaries and extra coverage during training sessions which could also mean overtime pay.

You need to decide who needs training and how to manage the cost-benefit ratio, i.e. should you buy the film or share it with other companies in the area? Should you ignore the requirement and hope to not get investigated? How can you decide and what should be done? OSHA believes transit personnel are at risk even though your drivers report an incidence of vomiting or injury about once every six months.

5. At a recent workshop for the mass transit industry, workman's compensation cases were discussed. Lately 3 persons filed and won compensation for heart attacks on the basis of their having a high stress job. This was in spite of the fact that they participated in high risk behaviors like smoking and drinking a lot of coffee. These were all top level managers and were very productive and creative people.

The parent company is concerned because of the steep rise in workman's compensation insurance and because the public relations manager of the parent company had a heart attack last year. For a while there was reportedly careful diet compliance and no smoking but recently these behaviors have returned. The top administrators of the parent company are considering finding a way to force resignation of this public relations manager. Your division has been asked to file a confidential report of agreement or non-agreement to the forced retirement and why you hold that position.

APPENDIX E:
COMMENTARY ON SELECT CONVERSATION
STARTERS AND REFLECTION SUBMISSIONS

The following are selected conversation starter and reflection submission questions from the chapters along with sample answers written in italics.

Chapter 1:
Conversation Starters: *One can see these questions can be answered in a common-sense way.*

4. Support your reasoning that we, as a community, should or should not fund speculative scientific projects. *Scientific projects are just one potential community funding decision. Opening parks could be another, but in the chapter we discussed scientific projects.*

   a. *One could argue yes to fund projects because of the many helpful products that came from the space mission research.*

   b. *One could argue no because of the millions of people, especially children who die from insufficient food and clean water in underdeveloped countries.*

   c. *It can be argued that just because we can do something does not mean we ought to do it.*

Reflection-submissions:

1. Can one's cultural heritage lead to immoral actions? Provide an example where culture provides positive guidance then provide an example of culture not leading positively. By what standard (standards) did you make this evaluation? *The purpose of this activity is for students to be sensitive to their bias towards the way they do things. Positive tradition would be sending children to school; not positive would be female genital mutilation and some other tribal rites of passage. Usually, this evaluation would be based on the student's own culture. "It must be right because we do it."*

2. Write a reflection sharing your ideas and experiences of situations in which values made a difference. Explain why you say what you say about the situations. Share your understanding of the

connections between values and actions. *With these reflections, students have submitted a wide variety of experiences. The desire is for students to thoughtfully consider the impact of values.*

Chapter 2:
Conversation Starters:
4. How does one learn what another person values? List some values which make a difference in how people are treated? *The point of this item is that we cannot know what the other person values without asking them. We usually assume our friends, even our acquaintances with similar appearances, share the same values. Values which make a difference in how people are treated include: body size, being athletic, being without apparent disability, skin and hair color.*

5. Use examples and arguments to support or refute the position that respecting human dignity is the normative principle for how we ought to treat people? You will need to begin by providing what you think "respecting human dignity" means. *Suggested content: "Respecting human dignity" means respecting the choices other persons make because human dignity is based on unique human capacities of reason and will, which is freedom of choice based on knowledge. This is the concept of autonomy. For example, mocking religious views is to be avoided. Disrespecting persons of different views violates their dignity. Example of reasoning: this crowd is gathering to protest differences of religion. This protest violates human dignity, so, I cannot participate. This successful use of human dignity argues for its normative value, perhaps not definitively.*

Reflection Submissions:
1. Write a practical syllogism to resolve a situation of moral tension. Do this as if you were the one who needed to act. *The example in 3 above is an example for this. This crowd is gathering to protest differences of religion. This protest violates human dignity, so, I cannot participate. Another example might be: Giving donations to street panhandlers encourages them to remain homeless, the person on the corner is asking for donations, I cannot contribute because remaining homeless is not safe. (Content not meant to assert a position on contributions to the poor.)*

Chapter 3:
Conversation Starters:

3. Discuss the following with two or three classmates: Does Aristotle or Plato's position on the nature of existence seem stronger to you? Prepare a group response in the form of argument (s) using this content and life experiences. Prepare assertive sentences s premises concluding to the chosen position. *The main purpose of this assignment is to have students writing arguments. There is no right answer beyond the provision of premises that account for the selected conclusion. The summaries are in Chapter 3 Conversation Starter 1.*

Reflection submissions:

3. From reading Plato and Aristotle, including the Discussion Starter Chapter 3-1, do humans have souls dwelling in bodies or souls united to the materials of the body. Support your answer. *Students divide in seeing humans as souls within bodies and body-soul unities. The goal is to think about this deep question. The ancient philosophers used soul to mean principle of life. Today so many of us think of spirituality when we hear the word soul. Either Plato or Aristotle believed in a personal God. Plato's content refers to an ultimate place of perfections. In Plato origins and sustenance are within the Form of the Good. Aristotle wants a naturalistic explanation, but at the end of the Physics, he argues that at the outermost sphere of the universe there is an ultimate being which draws all to itself through an indifferent love, agape. Philosophy can provide proofs for ultimate being, but cannot tell us more.*

4. Animals like birds and mammals have to shelter from the heat, cold, rain and sun. Bird nests are said to be by nature because each kind of bird builds the same nest as all other birds of that kind. Considering human shelters, what about the shelter is natural and what is artificial. Be sure to begin with definitions of these terms. *To need shelter is natural for humans. The materials may be natural, if wood or earth. The design is an artifact of human creativity and some building materials are artifacts. It may be argued that it is natural of humans to design their shelter and thus the structure is natural. It is by convention that what a human makes is called artificial and what a bird makes is called natural. This is called the natural-artificial distinction.*

Chapter 4:
Conversation Starters:
1. Define concepts and provide examples of concepts that remain the same and concepts that are ever changing. *Concepts are certainly not the ever-changing material world. For example, the concept or idea of requiring shelter remains the same. The shelter provided by humans changes by materials available, location, custom, and time in history.*
2. We say human persons are to be treated with respect. Yet this does not always happen.
   a. Describe a time when you clearly felt you were being treated as a person.
   b. Describe a time when you clearly felt you were being treated as a thing. What could have been done to transform this situation into one with you feeling like a person. *This discussion assists students to make a clear distinction in behavior that is respectful and what is not. A recalled example from a student paper was feeling special and of worth when being recruited, but feeling like a thing when the student was injured and unable to perform as the coach had expected. What could have made a difference is if the coach could have seen beyond the game to the players as humans valued for themselves as well as their performance.*

Reflection Submissions:
4. Provide your answer and use arguments to support your position, why do humans exist? What is the end or purpose of human life? *This reflects Victor Frankl that one needs a goal or purpose to make life meaningful. But one can still ask, must there be an overarching purpose as well as individual perspectives. Why humanity? I'm sure you recognize this is the most important question one can answer, why are we here?*

Chapter 5:
Conversation Starters:
4. Is not telling the truth you know different from lying to cover over the truth you know. Describe a time, if any, when it's right to lie. Identify a time, if any, when it's right to not tell the truth. Is there a value higher than truth-telling? *This can be very difficult because conscientious people often hold one ought never to lie, and I would agree with this ordinarily. In caring for others, providers are often not allowed to disclose what they know about patient*

conditions and laboratory data. Rather than abruptly declare, I cannot tell you, many professionals will return the question with a question about the concern behind the question, "what do you think" or "what is on your mind?" Telling the truth often opposes the moral principle to do no harm.

Reflection Submissions:

2. Consideration of student's disciplinary code of ethics: Obtain a copy of the Code of Ethics for a health-care discipline of your choice. These are available on-line by looking for the code of ethics for your discipline or one closely related. Write short answers and support for your answers to the following questions (using in your paper specific items from your code as evidence):

   a.) Does it include your relationship with other members of the profession?

   b.) Does it provide for the continuance of the discipline?

   c.) Does it address what treatment is within the purview of the discipline?

   d.) What are the dominant themes and positions promoted in the code?

   e.) Does it address human rights? In what way?

   f.) Does it provide content needed to resolve an ethical situation into an optimum action?

   Support your answers.

Just a couple notes, (c) is not usually addressed in codes of ethics. This is directed by state or county practice acts for the discipline. Thinking about (f), codes provide guidance. They do not resolve specific ethical questions. This requires practitioners with knowledge of principles, policies and codes that can be applied within specific situations to come to a decision on the ethical thing to be done.

Chapter 6:

Conversation Starters:

4. Describe what you would do if you saw a conflict between hospital policy and one of the standards of human rights? *It would seem important that one work toward changing hospital policy. The first step would be to bring this to the attention of one's supervisor. If you are ignored or even ridiculed you would need to speak with the next higher person, like head of your department. It is not advisable to bring this to the public press unless you have taken the item all the way to the chief executive officer, or highest administrator and feel called to notify the public because you*

judge there is severe risk to patients. Be sure you are not just interested in the acknowledgement as whistleblowers often pay a serious price for their efforts.

Reflection Submissions:

2. Obtain a copy of your disciplinary code of ethics. Write a short paper of how your codes are similar and different from the Universal Declaration of Human Rights, and either the Nuremburg Codes or the Helsinki Accords. *This could be quite simply answered by students that they contain similar ideas but the Nuremberg and Helsinki Declarations address research situations.*

Chapter 7:

Conversation Starters:

2. In your best judgment, what is required for a community to be at peace? Will this ever be achieved in the family? The health facility? Or, in society? *An abundance of respect for others, virtue and love. This is more common within the family because of the foundation in love. The diversity of values and customs makes peace more difficult in the work place or society at large.*

Reflection Submissions:

4. Use Mr. JD and the framework provided as an example to resolve and write out a sample dilemma in your discipline, your life, or being in school. Use situations with issues other than confidentiality. *Students tend to just copy the JD discussion in another situation of confidentiality, like telling the coach a friend is drinking before a game. This prevents them gaining the experience of thinking through the process as intended. This is worth being a major assignment for the course.*

5. **Part one:** Augustine would consider the higher value to be the more immaterial option. What would Augustine say about the following:

Suggestions are my best thought. As always, there are other options.

   a. Having sufficient food and shelter or receiving free tuition *Free tuition seems material but allows for leaning, which is immaterial, so I take this item.*

   b. Having the freedom to attend the school of your choice or graduating from college without debt *While one would not want to choose not to have knowledge in order to stay debt free, being thus leaves one free to choose location and type of employment.*

    c. Graduating from college without debt or being respected in the community *Respect is likely a higher value than being debt free because it is a very immaterial facet of human life.*

    d. Receiving respect from family or from a health-care provider *Probably family because grounded on love and source of personal values.*

    e. Having good health or virtue *definitely virtue as the excellence of soul.*

    f. Doing satisfying work or controlling your own schedule *Debatable, but seems to involve more thoughtfulness.*

    g. Being in a beautiful environment or listening to beautiful music *The environment is more holistic.*

Part two: Rank the above Reflection options (1 a – g) based on your values and support your choices. Explain your answers, supporting your choices.

Chapter 8
Conversation Starters:

2. It has often been argued that if you were starving or if you had starving children at home, it would be moral for you to steal food, or take a loan you know you will not be able to repay because life is the higher value. What would Kant say? Share your reasoning on his behalf using the Categorical Imperative and the foundation in how rational beings ought to be treated. Consider especially what taking the food or money says about the grocer or banker from whom the items are taken. *Kant holds one may reason like this in normal self-oriented thinking but considering the categorical imperative one cannot wish that all persons steal or lie to get what they want or even need as this would collapse the economic system. Additionally, these behaviors treat others as a means to your end and not as ends in themselves, which is Kant's requirement.*

Reflection Submissions:

4. Explain why you would choose to be taken care of by someone who focused on justice and rights-based care or someone who focused on relational caring-based care. *Just let me note that we usually want someone to care for us who has an empathetic heart and makes care-based decisions. When we are not receiving the loyalty of a caring, relational person, or when policies are being made, we want persons to be justice and rights- based.*

Chapter 9
Conversation Starters:

7. What about the little one changes at birth that provides the right to life? Given that the fetus can be legally killed, even in the birth canal, this seems to be the moment of acquiring rights. Support your answers with premises from science and reason. *This is a common issue in discussions at the beginning of life. Nonetheless, there are few good answers. Because of C-section births, it is admitted that traversing the birth canal does not confer humanity on the newborn. There are religious communities which hold human life begins with the first breath. They reference Genesis where it says, God breathed on Adam and he became a living soul. Evidence from science points to human genome activation 52 hours after the sperm reaches the ovum because the cell which activates becomes the body of the embryo and guides development of the new human. On the contrary, scientists doing research on the cellular embryo consider it a human embryo but not human. (This does not seem to be what I meant to say, but it is what is said.) You are invited to read the discussion of George and Lee, n. 140.*

Reflection Submissions:

4. This is a good time for you to assert a position when human life begins and when moral rights are attributed to the new individual, include rationales for your position. What difference does it make? Write your thoughts on each of the following: Would your view on abortion, cloning, or embryonic stem cell research change given each of the following possibilities?

    e. What if there is no immaterial soul, the mind is an expression of biochemical function, sometimes called epiphenomena?

    f. What if the individual is an expression of the evolutionary process?

    g. What if the individual comes into existence with a soul from an ultimate immaterial source?

    h. What if an ultimate being did design the universe but has no further involvement in human life?

This work has resulted in fruitful classroom discussions. Sometimes the four positions have been placed on the board with questions of the impact on valuing of the community, individual or group; the unborn; the disabled. Item c is explanatory for why some religious groups value each human. No matter how young and undeveloped, they are a child of God.

Chapter 10
Conversation Starters:

6. If you were assigned to care for a patient from whom medical nutrition and hydration have been withdrawn? Would you be complicit in the person's death because you are caring for them? Support your answer. *This question recalls our early discussion of implied consent. You know they are not receiving food and fluid. By your presence you assert your approval. In your discomfort you may be complaining to colleagues. It depends on your practice; some practitioners can ask for evaluation and suggestions from the Ethics Committee. Using the principle of double effect, one may consider if withdrawal of food and fluids was to prevent fluid overload at the end of life or if the intent is to have the patient die. Could this be letting the patient die?*

Reflection Submissions:

1. To a great extent, decisions of whether or not to feed someone at the end of their life have been related to religious perspectives. Setting religious reasons aside, what leads to the requirement of providing food and fluid when the patient no longer feeds themselves? What argues we do not need to provide food and fluid in these same circumstances? Provide an argument from ethical principles for your personal position for or against providing food and fluids. *This item is asking for respect of human dignity and use of science. With knowledge determining if the patient is in their last days or not, and knowledge of end of life responses to food and fluids one can act to do no harm.*

Chapter 11
Conversation Starters:

2. You are on the admissions board of a prominent university. A 19-year-old with conviction of burglary and theft at age 16 is applying for admission as a prelaw student. You have had the experience of admitting a student with a police record before. They completed at the university, even law school, then were not allowed to sit for the Bar exam. Reportedly, there was a question if they met the character requirements. Provide answers and principle-based reasons for your decisions. *It may seem peculiar to use a situation related to law school versus a health-care example, but the idea is to consider the activities and rights of a profession as a self-governing body.*

   a. Ought professions be allowed to restrict someone capable of the academic work? *In practice, this is done and it seems right because a professional has a special calling in the community. There are character requirements that protect the profession itself and individuals not emotionally suited to the practices of the profession. Comparable are requirements that sex offenders not be teachers.*

b. Would you recommend the person for regular admission or provisional admission to the university? *There is no reason for this person's legal record to impact their admission to the university. It seems a violation of privacy that this information is even involved in the admission question, whether it comes from public record or personal contacts. The concerned party may want to share his experience and suggest the student seek a different major, but only if this person's legal record is public knowledge.*

c. Does the admissions committee have a responsibility to question this admission? *No. Each person deserves an education. This person's past record will be reviewed by a profession's governing board. Within professional licensure in health care one is asked about felony convictions. This may impact licensure. There are areas within the legal and health professions where one with a legal record could, theoretically find employment. Career counselors need to be aware of these issues.*

Reflection Submissions:

1. Provide arguments to show health-care is a right, or that it is not a right but a human need that people ought to fulfill for themselves? Support your answer. *Let me develop an argument for health care being a right: (1) The Declaration of Independence holds that all persons have the right to life, (2) a long and productive life requires good health, (3) good health requires regular attendance by health professionals, and thus it can be argued that health-care is a right. Alternately, one could argue that the right to life is limited to not killing you rather than caring for you and the kind of life you have.*

GLOSSARY

Glossary Entry	Definition	Chapter
accidental	attributes which do not follow on the kind of being under consideration but secondary to its being a particular kind.	4
active euthanasia	end-of-life interventions that kill with or without consent.	10
analogical	meaning that some aspects vary and some stay the same. Provides new understandings for research, and according to Aquinas allows humans to grasp a bit of Divine meanings like love.	2
analogical reasoning	ethical inquiry based on similarities and differences between historic cases and the current situation.	7
antecedent	the "if" portion of a hypothetical statement.	3
Argument	A set of claims, one of which is the conclusion the others are support for the conclusion called premises.	2
Aristotelian form	An internal principle of activity and rest that makes something that exists be what it is.	3
artificial	human made, having its principle of change imposed from the outside.	3
attributed dignity	value and worth added by respect of the community from what one has done.	2
Autonomy	One of the principles of the ethical theory of Principlism indicating respect for self-determination.	2 and 8
autonomy	Respect for personal choices that were based on knowledge.	2
Beneficence	the long term good.	2 and 8
brain death	loss of function of the whole brain as integrating organ of the body.	9 and 10

brute	in Aristotle this person is unable to make moral decisions because of a lack of ability to understand.	7
caring	actions that include tenderness, careful performance of duties, or use of good judgment.	5
Categorical Imperative	the moral perspective of Kant, one ought to act as if the maxim of behavior would become a universal law of nature.	8
civil rights	these rights are secured by law, the legal norms of a community or country.	11
claim	An assertive sentence.	2
clinical death	irreversible loss of respiration and circulation.	9 and 10
cogitative sense	a protective response of the inner senses in collaboration with human.	4
coma	loss of consciousness, may be temporary or permanent.	10
comfort feeding	an end of life approach that spoon feeds the patient only what they want to eat.	10
communion	The union of individual persons moving towards others which leads to the formation of community.	4
concept	An idea formed in the mind, immaterial and universal.	2
Conclusion	A claim of an argument which asserts that which is supported within the argument.	2
conscientious objection	asking for exception to protect one's conscience.	6
consequent	the "then" portion of a hypothetical statement.	3
consequentialism	in ethical decisions gives priority to anticipated outcomes, only outcomes carry value.	7
cost/benefit analysis	consideration of actual and social costs balanced against beneficial outcomes.	11
Courage	one of the four cardinal virtues that gives strength to act on the known proper behavior.	7
decision-making capacity	a formal determination of the patient's ability to know, understand and decide their own interventions.	10

deductive	reasoning from generalizations to other generalizations or specific cases.	2
dignity	to have internal and social worth.	2
Equality	Valuing and treating each human equally.	1
equity	distribution of goods and services according to actual or potential contribution.	11
equivocal	a term with more than one meaning. This variance leads to equivocation, which can nullify an argument. The source of much humor.	2
essential	Attributes which follow on the kind of being under consideration (characteristic of the kind).	4
estimative	refers to one of the inner senses in an animal that leads to attraction or repulsion as an automatic response.	4
Ethic of Care	finds moral guidance from within the web of relationships inherent in each ethical situation.	8
Ethical Dilemma	a conflict of values, policies, or principles so that one must determine priorities among them. A person can only do one of the two possible actions and once you have acted you cannot go back and undo what was done.	2 and 7
Ethics	Study of proper human behavior.	1
extraordinary care	interventions which are not well established, not readily available, nor affordable, and associated with great suffering.	4
fallacy	An Invalid argument form that looks like a secure argument following the valid formal argument but is not.	3
fallacy of affirming antecedent	An Invalid argument form that looks like the valid Modus Ponens argument.	3
fallacy of denying consequent	An invalid argument form that looks like the valid Modus Tollens argument.	3
form	that which makes something be 'what it is'.	3
Harvard Criteria	the standard of brain death since 1968 accepted as death in all 50 states.	10

healing act	Exchange between individuals in which one person is enriched in their quest for health by the presence and abilities of another.	5
health	a state of excellence with the proper functioning of the inorganic, vegetative, sensitive and intellectual capacities.	4
health-care arts	application of principles within situations, clinical practice and ethics are examples.	5
health-care organizations	communities, relational social systems, whose proper end or goal is increasing the health of those who come within the organization's care as patients, clients, or employees.	11
health-care science	a stable base of organized knowledge generated by documented controlled inquiry.	5
Hippocratic tradition	the physician is responsible to tell the patient the best course of action for their situation.	8
hominization	a technical philosophical term for embryonic reception of a human intellectual soul.	9
human act	action chosen and freely carried out as one's own.	5
hypothetical	if…then reasoning.	3
hypothetical imperative	what you must do to achieve something.	8
ideal person	for Aristotle this is what one ought to aim for to have a peaceful happy life, the fullness of all human goods.	7
iff	abbreviation for indicating in a hypothetical argument, if and only if the antecedent will the consequent follow.	3
immaterial	without matter, cannot be sensed, but can be known.	2
implied consent	one's association with a situation is one's assent to what is occurring.	9
individuation	the time beyond which the embryo can no longer be twins.	9
inductive	reasoning from particulars of experience to generalizations.	2

informed consent	A freely chosen approval given for admission to a facility or treatment with knowledge of options.	4
inner senses	these receive nerve impulses from stimuli in the environment and form them into an image (phantasm).	4
integrity	a person of integrity has personal and professional values integrated with public works.	11
intellect	the human capacity to abstract universal content as concepts, form propositions and to judge them true or false.	4
interpersonal system	The space where practitioner, patient and family enter into dialogue and interaction.	4
intrinsic dignity	a deep value or worth from the kind of being one is.	2
Justice	Ultimate Platonic Form for excellence in personal and interpersonal affairs leading to inner peace and happiness. It is also one of the pillars of Principlism.	5 and 8
justice	Human excellence of treating others with fairness, and proper distribution of goods and services.	5
knowing	To have the presence of the object of thought in the mind of the knower.	3
locked-in syndrome	lack of communication between hemispheres of the brain and spinal nerves.	10
logic	the tool of the intellect that prepares the mind for clear systematic thinking and for analyzing arguments	2
material	exists as solid, can be sensed, and confined as matter.	2
matter	is that 'out of which' something is made.	3
metaphysics	the division of philosophy that searches into the origins and principles of existence.	2
modally distinct	means that we can separate items when we think about them, but they are not actually separate.	4
Moderation	one of the four cardinal virtues, the virtue of self-discipline.	7

Modus Ponens	a valid logical form of hypothetical argument, if p, then q: and p, therefore q.	3
ModusTollens	A valid form of hypothetical argument, if p, then q: and not q, therefore not p.	3
Moral	your own values and principles that operationalize these values.	1
moral act	excellent human action that moves the person or community towards the human good.	5
moral maxim	an applicable principle, an ought.	2
morality	an individual's principles and values that form a basis of action.	8
natural philosophy	the division of philosophy that studies the changeable world, matter in motion. Includes what we call today the natural sciences, ethics and politics.	2
natural rights	these rights are secured by the kind of being humans; life, liberty and the pursuit of happiness.	11
naturally moral person	inclined by nature to see and do what ought to be done in all situations.	7
nature	A term for either the world around us or the inner force that brings something to be what it is, the form.	3
Nonmaleficence	to do no harm.	2 and 8
normative	ethical reasoning based on norms or principles.	2 and 8
ordinary care	interventions which are well established, readily available, affordable and not associated with great suffering.	4
outer senses	these receive stimuli from the environment and communicate the nerve impulses to inner senses.	4
passive euthanasia	end-of-life interventions that remove medical equipment that are preventing death.	10
paternalism	An approach to patients that assumes the health-care provider knows what is best.	4
percept	that which is developed as a consequence of the process of perception.	4

Persistent Vegetative State (PVS)	A comatose state lasting for an extended period of time.	**3 and 10**
person	an individual substance of a relational nature - Boethius.	**6**
personal being	one in charge of its own life, self-governing (Boethius).	**4**
personal system	the core of health-care captures the substantial physical individual, body and soul.	**4**
philosophical	The tendency to question and desire precise answers about the nature of existence.	**2**
philosophy	The love of wisdom.	**2**
Platonic Forms	Eternal Perfections outside the world of change.	**3**
potential	the capacity to be that which it is not yet.	**3**
practical reasoning	application of principles within situations, clinical practice and ethics are examples.	**2**
practical syllogism	reasoning that applies a moral principle within a situation. The conclusion is that this situation is or is not a case of the principle. As a syllogism there are three claims: principle, situation and conclusion, which is what ought to be done.	**2**
practical wisdom	the ability to act on one's moral decision. This is also called prudence.	**2**
Premise	A claim which provides support for the conclusion in an argument.	**2**
principle of double effect	an undesirable second effect is morally tolerable if the good end is intended and the secondary effect is not the cause of the good end. The good must be sufficiently good to validate the tolerance of evil.	**9**
principle of identity	Whatever is is, a tautology.	**2**
principle of individuation	matter in its ability to set apart individuals.	**3**
principle of non-contradiction	First principle of reasoning. The same thing cannot both be and not be at the same time in the same respect.	**2**

sound argument	a deductively valid argument with true premises.	2
stem cell	a type of reserved cell in cord blood, fat, skin and mammary glands available to grow and repair tissues.	9
strong-willed person	knows what ought to be done, makes the decision to do so and does the good.	7
substance	Natural or artificial items in our world of change that are matter/form unities.	3
substantial form	an internal force that is stabilizing, unifying and specifying, it makes an individual be what it is.	3
substantiality	being-in-itself, with an inner-privacy and the potential for self-transcendence and self-conscious awareness.	4
substantial	Refers to humans being Aristotelian matter/form substances.	4
syllogism	a formal argument with three claims. Evaluation of strength or validity is dependent on the relationships between the subject and predicate terms and a middle term that connects the others.	2
tautology	a general statement which cannot be false, like all that is is.	2
truth	as something is. The object in the mind corresponds to the object outside of the mind.	2
truth	when the known object in the intellect is the same as the item in the world outside of the intellect.	4
universal	outside of space and time, immaterial like concept.	2
univocal	a term that has the same meaning every time it is used.	2
Utilitarianism	proposes evaluation and decision making based on agreeable consequences.	8
valid argument	relationship between the terms of the premises secure that if the premises are true the conclusion must be true.	2
Value	That which is treasured.	1
vicious	an evil person who rationalizes to allow whatever is desired.	7
virtue	an excellence of the soul.	4

principle of stability	that which is shared by all things specified as the same kind.	3
Principlism	the position that there are four pillars of ethical behavior in health settings, Nonmaleficence, Beneficence, Autonomy and Justice.	2 and 8
professional	a person set aside by society to fulfill necessary roles within the community.	5
Proposition	Assertions or affirmative sentences that can be premises and or conclusions in an argument. Also called claims.	2
prudence	the ability to act on one's moral decision. It is also called practical wisdom.	2
rationality	the intellectual ability to reason with immaterial concepts.	9
relational	the phenomenal capacity of humans to be for others.	4
relationality	The tendency of humans to move beyond themselves into communion with others.	4
relativism	ethical reasoning based on the idea the situation determines what ought to be done not norms or principles.	2
responsibilities	reciprocal to rights, ones duties because of certain rights or ones position in community.	6
rights	protections and entitlements.	6
science	seeking knowledge of nature through a precise inquiry.	2
self-consciousness	Human self-awareness or self-presence, that is, an objective distance providing awareness of one's self both as present to one's self and others and as the source of one's actions.	4
self-defense argument	it is acceptable to take a person's life if they are threatening your life.	9
Glossary Entry	**Definition**	**Cha**
self-transcendence	an over-flowing of the inner-self towards others characteristic of rational being.	4
social system	characterizes all health-care settings, including transcendent health-care activities.	4

vulnerable	incapable of protecting one's own interest.	6
weak-willed person	knows what ought to be done and makes the decision to do so but at last moment does the desired evil.	7
will	desire for the known generated in the knower by what is known.	4
Wisdom	one of the four cardinal virtues, the virtue of good judgment, knowing what ought to be done.	7